S0-ACP-100

LEGENDARY CHINESE HEALING HERBS

Henry C. Lu

 Sterling Publishing Co., Inc.   New York

Edited by Laurel Ornitz

Library of Congress Cataloging-in-Publication Data

Lu, Henry C.
    Legendary Chinese healing herbs / Henry C. Lu.
        p.   cm.
    Includes index.
    ISBN 0-8069-8230-6
    1. Herbs—Therapeutic use.   2. Medicine, Chinese.   I. Title.
RM666.H33L76   1991
615'.321'0951—dc20   90-24290
                                                      CIP

10 9 8 7 6 5 4 3 2 1

Contents

Preface

There are no fabulous stories about ordinary herbs, just as there are no fabulous stories about ordinary people. For people to become legendary figures, they must be heroic or outstanding in some way. For herbs to achieve legendary status, they must be considered to be extraordinarily effective. There are, all in all, over 5,000 Chinese herbs, but only a fraction of them have made their way to becoming celebrated herbs in Chinese legends. These are the herbs that have been traditionally regarded by the Chinese people to be most effective and useful in their quest for freedom from disease and in their maintenance of good health.

I'm sure you will enjoy these stories, although some are undoubtedly more interesting or amusing than others. Eventually, however, you will most likely move beyond the sphere of mere enjoyment, as you come to realize through personal experience or theoretical understanding that these legendary herbs still play an important role in the promotion of health today. On my part, interesting though it is to tell fabulous stories about Chinese herbs, I had a more serious intent in mind in writing this book, which was to make people more keenly aware of the existence of these exceptional herbs and to tell them how they can make use of them in promoting their own health. In this sense, this book is more than a collection of legends about Chinese herbs—it is a practical guide to Chinese herbs for natural health by natural means.

In the prehistoric period, before the written language was invented, the Chinese people could only communicate verbally, and in order to hand down their knowledge about herbs to their posterity, they had to rely on telling stories. In order to create deeper impressions in their listeners, the stories about herbs were not confined to their effects and uses, but often included episodes about how they had initially been discovered and what tragedies or comedies and heroism were involved. As with other kinds of stories, many of these stories about herbs had fictitious events, making them like fairy tales, to catch the attention of the listeners. As time went on, such stories became legends, and the herbs became legendary herbs in the history of Chinese herbalism.

From the point of view of pharmacology, the legends about Chinese herbs cannot be used as data for research into the effects of herbs, because

5

legends are no more than unverifiable stories handed down by tradition from earlier times, and many of them are full of myths and fabrications. On the other hand, it is a fact that virtually all the stories reveal effects of herbs that are consistent with those commonly recognized by professional Chinese herbalists, both past and present. For example, in the story about puff balls, the herb was depicted as an outstanding herb to use for the arrestment of bleeding, and in modern Chinese herbalism, this same herb is still used for this purpose. In another story, Siberian motherwort was described as a wonder herb for mothers, and in modern Chinese herbalism, it is still regarded as an important herb for women's ailments, such as irregular menstruation, menstrual pain, disorders associated with childbirth, and numerous other female symptoms.

Most of the stories about the herbs are relatively short and are characterized by literary simplicity. But, nevertheless, all of them reflect very well and sometimes poignantly the important uses of the particular herbs.

In addition to the herbs and their legends, this book includes descriptions of the 20 major classifications of herbs. The herbs represent all these classifications. This is by no means a mere coincidence, because the herbs included here are all important herbs and can even be considered the elite group of Chinese herbs, and as such, it is natural for them to stand out distinctly in the various classifications.

It is important for you to know about at least one herb in each of the 20 classifications, because the herbs in each are the best for treating a particular group of symptoms. For example, diseases associated with inflammation and infection are as a general rule treated by those herbs that reduce excessive heat inside the body, and if you are familiar with at least one herb in this class, you will be able to make effective use of it whenever you are troubled by inflammation or infection. Herbs that reduce heat inside the body are one of the most important classes of herbs, which is why a number of herbs presented in this book fall under this classification.

Some of the herbs in this book can also be considered Western herbs in the sense that either they are readily available in many natural foods stores and are familiar to Western people in general, or they are frequently used by Western herbalists in their clinical practice. Such "Western" herbs include agrimony, black false hellebore, boneset, Chinese ephedra, danggui, garlic, jimson weed, Korean mint, kudzu vine, licorice, mistletoe, purslane, and rhubarb. As to the exclusively Chinese herbs, all of them are available in any Chinese herb shop. On an average, these shops stock more than 1,000 herbs in dried form. The vast majority of Chinese herbs are available in dried form for decoction, not because of convenience or economy, but because dried herbs contain very little water, which is not a necessary ingredient and may even decrease the effects of certain herbs. Since my intention is not merely to entertain my readers, but also to benefit them in their quest for good health, the availability of the herbs included in this book makes its contents all the more relevant.

6

In China today, Chinese and Western medicine are practised side by side, and a patient has a choice between the two types of medicine. However, a mindful patient will always make use of both types of medicine to his or her best advantage. And the reader is reminded that in case of illness, it is always wise to consult a qualified physician to ensure that he or she gets the best possible medical care available in modern society.

Introduction

There are four basic branches of Chinese medicine: Chinese herbalism, Chinese food cures, Chinese acupuncture, and Chinese manipulative therapy. In most instances, a Chinese physician will be more likely to practise these four branches of Chinese medicine simultaneously, but various branches may also be practised separately in different clinics.

In general, however, Chinese herbalism and Chinese food cures are almost always practised together. Likewise, it is also customary for an acupuncturist to practise manipulative therapy as well, but today in China one can also see manipulative therapy set up as a separate department in hospitals the same way as acupuncture. Broadly speaking, traditional Chinese medicine can be divided into internal medicine, which includes herbalism and food cures, and external medicine, which includes acupuncture and manipulative therapy as well as other external treatment techniques such as moxibustion, acupressure, ironing, and cupping.

THE ORIGINS OF CHINESE MEDICINE

From the remains excavated in China by archaeologists, primitive people are believed to have inhabited the Chinese mainland as far back as 600,000 or even one million years ago. For instance, the fossil remains of Peking man found in a cave at Choukoutien near Peking have been identified as belonging to the Pleistocene epoch that originated about a million years ago.

These primitive people had to work and find food, and they had to take steps to prevent the attack of disease or to cure it. Therefore, some sort of medicine or health care was a necessity among the primitive people in their struggle for survival, which marked the beginning of traditional Chinese medicine in the prehistorical period.

In the process of finding food, they must have mistakenly eaten poisonous foods from time to time that caused vomiting, diarrhea, or even death. It was from such experiences that they gradually came to identify the plants that were good as foods as well as those that were poisonous and could only be used to heal diseases.

A Chinese classic published in the West Han Dynasty (206 B.C.–A.D. 24),

9

entitled *Huai Nan Taoists,* relates a story about a Chinese emperor of agriculture in ancient China who was said to have tasted one hundred plants each day to determine whether they were suitable for human consumption. The emperor was said to have been poisoned over seventy times each day in the process. Although this emperor of agriculture may not have actually existed, the story is generally regarded as an indication of a society shifting from hunting to farming as a way of life, and the emperor is given credit for the origin of Chinese herbalism.

There is a Chinese saying that states, "One cannot always draw a line between foods and herbs." This is because some herbs (such as Asian dandelion and Chinese yam) are so mild in effect and so pleasing to the taste that they can be eaten as foods, and some foods (such as garlics, dried ginger, and red dates) also contain healing properties sufficiently powerful for them to be used as herbs. Thus, in Chinese medicine, many plants are considered both foods and herbs at the same time. And it's for this reason that food cures have always been practised side by side with Chinese herbalism, and Chinese physicians often make it a point to advise their patients to take certain herbs and eat certain foods simultaneously in order to cure an illness.

An ancient Chinese classic, entitled *Classic of Mountains and Water,* states, "Stone needles may be found on high mountains." This classic marked the beginning of Chinese acupuncture. Subsequently, bone needles, bamboo needles, and other types of needles have been invented for use in acupuncture treatment. This classic also pioneered in the development of Chinese herbalism in that it listed over 150 plants, 270 animals, and 64 minerals for medical uses.

As the primitive people in China tried to keep warm by fire, they gradually discovered that fire was able to heal many symptoms such as abdominal pain and pain in the joints (known as arthritis today). From such experiences, the Chinese arts of healing called moxibustion and ironing were originally discovered. Both of these types of therapy involve the use of heat and herbs simultaneously. The discovery of fire in China is considered to be a very significant event in the history of Chinese medicine, and it dates as far back as a half a million years ago when Peking man was said to have used fire for a variety of purposes.

Before the discovery of instruments in China, primitive people had to work with their hands, and when they got hurt and suffered from pain, they would instinctively attempt to heal their wounds and relieve their pain by touching the affected regions with the hands. As time went on, all of their experiences of healing wounds and relieving pain and curing other ailments by the use of hands accumulated, marking the beginning of Chinese manipulative therapy.

According to historians, the Chinese written language first came into existence during the so-called slave society between the twenty-first century B.C. and 476 B.C., and it significantly contributed to the development

10

of Chinese medicine. The transition from the slave society to the feudal society took place around the fifth century, B.C. During the feudal society (from 476 B.C. to 618 B.C.), major progress was made in virtually all aspects of Chinese culture, but most notably in politics, economics, and philosophy. It was during this period of history that different types of Chinese healing arts became integrated into a coherent system of medicine with the publication of *Nei Ching*, popularly known as the *Yellow Emperor's Classics of Internal Medicine*, which I translated into English in 1978. Any serious discussion of Chinese medicine must start with this first medical classic. In fact, the whole history of Chinese medicine can be said to be nothing more than a series of footnotes on this fundamental text.

It is worth mentioning that in terms of learning, a sharp contrast exists between Chinese and Western medicine. Students of Western medicine by and large consider learning the history of medicine to be little more than of historical interest because of its irrelevance to clinical practice, but students of Chinese medicine take medical classics very seriously because they are not only relevant but important to their clinical practice. For example, Richard Thomas Williamson (1862–1937), who invented the test for sugar in urine, is omitted from most contemporary Western medical dictionaries. One will also have great difficulty in finding the name of Friedrich Wilhelm Adam Sertuerner (1774–1841), a German pharmacist who isolated the active principle in opium called morphine, or the name of Caleb Hillier Parry (1755–1822), a British physician who identified one form of goiter called exophthalmic goiter.

On the other hand, any modern textbook on Chinese medicine will not fail to mention Shih-Chen Li, who wrote *An Outline of Materia Medica* in A.D. 1578, or Sun Shu Mao, who wrote *One Thousand Ounces of Gold Classic* in A.D. 652, because they are considered very important in the clinical practice of traditional Chinese medicine. How do we account for this sharp discrepancy between Chinese and Western medicine?

The use of an analogy may prove instructive. Learning Chinese medicine is like crossing a bridge whereas learning Western medicine is like building one. In learning how to build a new bridge, there is no need to know who had built what bridge centuries ago, for the knowledge established such a long time ago has become obsolete; but for someone learning how it feels to cross a bridge, the experiences of those who had crossed hundreds of bridges more than a thousand times many centuries ago are still very relevant and important. Knowledge about building bridges has continued to accumulate and improve day by day and new knowledge often proves to be the most effective, but there is also a risk, because the bridge built by new technology may collapse due to human error or incomplete knowledge. However, when it comes to medicine, the risk is increased considerably.

For example, in 1880 a Russian scientist conducted an experiment by feeding one group of lab rats fresh milk and other foods, and another group of lab rats the artificial products of pure protein, fats, carbohydrates, and minerals. His assumption was that the second group of lab rats would grow faster and become healthier because they had all the required nutrients for living and growing. But, as it turned out, the second group of lab rats died more quickly. What went wrong? The nutrients fed to the rats had been discovered by scientists to promote growth and improve health, so why did the rats die so quickly? The Russian scientist who conducted the experiment wrote, "There must be something missing which is physiologically indispensable but which has not been discovered."

Now we know that these lab rats were suffering from a deficiency of vitamins. But at that time, vitamins had not yet been discovered by scientists, who strongly believed that all a living creature needed was those nutrients already discovered and nothing else. The scientists didn't realize that their knowledge about nutrients was extremely limited and incredibly insufficient. Now one more type of nutrient called vitamins has been discovered, but what would happen if people were led to believe that all they needed were those nutrients alone and thus began to take the artificial products of those nutrients and nothing else? Western medicine is built on experimental knowledge, which often proves very effective but can also be very dangerous. As the saying goes, a little knowledge is a dangerous thing, which is a poignant description of the state of Western medicine.

On the other hand, Chinese medicine works more slowly but also more safely, which can be better in many cases; as the saying goes, it's better to be safe than sorry. Chinese medicine is based upon clinical experiences of many centuries and such experiences are as valid today as they were centuries ago. That is why Chinese physicians attach great importance to Chinese medical classics, which are the vital sources of experiences for them and are still relevant and important to clinical practice. It is for this reason that a student of Chinese medicine should make it a point to learn medical classics as thoroughly as possible. The authors of these medical classics had crossed hundreds of bridges over a thousand times, so to speak, and what they had to say represents their personal experiences of a lifetime spent as practitioners of Chinese medicine.

THE IMPORTANCE OF *NEI CHING* IN CHINESE MEDICINE

Although this classic has been attributed to the Yellow Emperor, most Chinese historians agree that the *Yellow Emperor's Classics of Internal Medicine (Nei Ching)* was not written by a single physician called the Yellow Emperor but by a group of Chinese physicians around the third century B.C. *Nei Ching* was not only a reflection of the medical achievements during that period of Chinese history, but it also established the fundamental principles underlying all aspects of Chinese medicine, becoming the ulti-

12

mate source for all subsequent developments. The theories outlined in this medical classic are still followed by Chinese physicians at the present time, virtually in the same way that Plato's philosophy is still admired by modern philosophers or the works of Shakespeare still revered by Western literary scholars.

The following is a passage from the *Yellow Emperor's Classics of Internal Medicine:* "A cold disease should be treated by hot herbs, and a hot disease should be treated by cold herbs." This principle of treatment is still considered valid today and is applied by virtually all Chinese physicians in their clinical practice. For example, goldthread, cork tree, and skullcap are all cold herbs, and for that reason, are used to treat hot disorders such as infectious and inflammatory illnesses, including mastitis, hepatitis, and enteritis. On the other hand, monkshood and dried ginger are both hot herbs, and are used to treat cold disorders such as cold sensations in the arms and legs, cold abdominal pain, cold arthritis and rheumatism, and cold diarrhea.

Another passage states, "Pungent and sweet herbs will disperse internal energy and they are yang herbs; sour and bitter herbs will cause diarrhea and they are yin herbs." This principle as well is still faithfully followed by Chinese physicians today. *Nei Ching* also states, "When a disease is confined to the superficial region, it should be treated by inducing perspiration." Today, a superficial disease such as the common cold or influenza is treated by the herbs for inducing perspiration.

In another connection, this classic says, "Energy is yang while flavour is yin," which is a concept still deemed valid today. For instance, it is a common principle in Chinese herbalism that the energy of herbs travels upwards and outwards and towards the skin and the arms and legs, which means that energy is yang, because yang travels upwards, outwards, and towards the skin and the arms and legs. Likewise, the flavor of herbs travels inward, downwards, and towards the internal organs, which means that flavor is yin, because yin travels inward, downwards, and towards the internal organs.

The Chinese system of food cures is also derived from *Nei Ching*. For example, a passage in the classic says, "One should eat cereal grains, meats, fruits, and vegetables properly in order to stay in good health." Another passage says, "When a person is ill, it may be necessary to treat the disease by herbs, but it is also necessary to eat five cereal grains as a principal nourishment, five fruits as a secondary nourishment, five animal meats to reinforce the energy, five vegetables to supplement deficiency, so that energy and flavour of foods will be combined to make the body stronger." This passage outlines the most fundamental food-cure principles in Chinese medicine.

Five cereal grains are rice, red beans, wheat and barley, soybeans, and broomcorn. Five fruits are peaches, pears, apricots, chestnuts, and red dates. Five animal meats are beef, lamb, pork, dog meat, and chicken. And five vegetables are vegetable marrow, leaves of pulse plants, scallions, green onions, and chives. This is a complete menu for good health because it contains virtually all the nutrients and in good proportion.

From the point of view of modern nutrition, cereal grains are the primary source of calories and proteins and also the source of vitamin B-complex and minerals; fruits are the primary source of vitamins and minerals; meats are the primary source of quality proteins and fats; and vegetables are the primary source of minerals, vitamins, and roughage. But, moreover, the passage in *Nei Ching* also proposes proportions of the different groups of foods that are consistent with the modern version of a healthy diet. In particular, both view eating more cereal grains than other groups of foods to be essential for good health.

In another connection, *Nei Ching* states, "When one suffers from kidney disease, one should refrain from eating huge amounts of salted foods" and "When a person consumes huge amounts of sweet foods and fatty foods, it may cause an accumulation of internal heat gradually turning into diabetes." This means, for example, that a patient with nephritis (which is an inflammation of the kidneys) should refrain from consumption of salt, and a diabetic should refrain from consumption of sugar. Both of these views are consistent with theories of modern nutrition.

In addition, the classic says, "It is necessary to attack diseases by internal consumption of herbs and also by external application of stone needles." This is a specific reference to treating disease with acupuncture. The theory of meridians outlined in *Nei Ching* still remains the most authoritative theory today, and all acupuncture students rely on this classic for valid information about meridians. As to the methods of treatment by acupuncture, the principles laid down in *Nei Ching* and upon which these methods are based are still faithfully adhered to by modern acupuncturists in both China and the West.

CHINESE HERBALISM CLASSICS

During the Chou Dynasty (1122–255 B.C.) as more herbs were being discovered and as the Chinese people were accumulating more experiences using herbs in the treatment of diseases, many Chinese publications were starting to mention herbs. For instance, the *Book of Rites*, published during this period, made mention of "five kinds of herbs," namely, grass, tree, worm, stone, and cereal, since the word "herb," as used in Chinese medicine, includes some animals and minerals, although the vast majority of Chinese herbs are plants.

When Chinese herbal therapy began to take shape, in around the fifth century, A.D., herbs were being discussed more extensively in books that also covered such subjects as astronomy and mathematics. But the first Chinese classic that exclusively dealt with herbs wasn't published until

14

prior to the East Han Dynasty (A.D. 25–220), and was attributed to the Emperor of Agriculture.

The *Classic of the Agriculture Emperor's Materia Medica*

This classic lists a total of 365 herbs, including 252 plants, 67 animals, and 46 minerals, which are each further divided into three classes. The upper class of herbs consists of herbs that are tonics and are either nontoxic or only slightly toxic, the middle class consists of herbs that are tonics with some effects of a therapeutic nature, and the lower class consists of mostly toxic herbs that are used exclusively for the treatment of disease. All in all, there are 120 herbs in the upper class, 120 herbs in the middle class, and 125 herbs in the lower class.

In addition, the *Classic of the Agriculture Emperor's Materia Medica* lists 170 diseases to be treated by herbs, including internal diseases, external diseases, women's diseases, diseases of the eyes, of the throat, of the ears, of the teeth, and so on. In many cases, the actions of herbs in the treatment of diseases, as set forth in this classic, are considered accurate and valuable today.

The original edition of the *Classic of the Agriculture Emperor's Materia Medica* was lost in the early years of the Tang Dynasty (A.D. 618–907), but its contents were retained in books published thereafter in the course of Chinese history. The People's Health Press in Peking published an edition of this classic in 1979 on the basis of data retained in other Chinese classics.

An Outline of Materia Medica

An Outline of Materia Medica was written by Shih-Chen Li (1518–1593) and published in 1578. In order to write this classic, the author was said to have read numerous Chinese classics and to have travelled extensively in order to identify the shapes of plants and the locations where they could be grown or found. Shi-Chen Li made great advances in the scrutiny of herbs as well as in their classifications. He classified all herbs into 16 categories, including water, fire, earth, metal-stone, grass, cereal, vegetable, fruit, tree, appliances, insect, scale, shell, domestic animal, bird, and man. Each category he further classified into subcategories. For instance, the category of grass was divided into 11 subcategories, including grass of mountains, aromatic grass, and marsh grass, and the category of tree was divided into six subcategories, including aromatic tree, tall tree, and shrub. Within the 16 categories, there were a total of 62 subcategories.

The entire classic contains approximately 1,900,000 Chinese ideograms and a list of 1,892 herbs, of which 374 the author added himself. Also included in this classic are 11,096 herbal formulas, which was the quadruple of what had previously been written by other authors. Many of these formulas are still considered extremely valuable today. The book also contains a total of 1,110 pictures of herbs.

15

In his classic, Shih-Chen Li adopted a more advanced method of classifying herbs. Virtually all Chinese herbalists in Li's time had made use of the upper, middle, and lower classifications of herbs, but Li destroyed this theory by classifying herbs in terms of plants, animals, and minerals, which is consistent with modern science and was a significant advance in the history of Chinese herbalism.

Another important step taken by Li in this classic was his division of herbs into families. For example, Peking cat thistle (Euphorbia pekinensis Rupr.), spurge (Euphorbia helioscopia L.), and caper spurge (Euphorbia lathyris L.) all have white juices in their stalks, and for that reason, Li classified all of them under the euphorbiaceae (spurge) family, which was indeed a scientific approach in line with modern botany.

One must remember in this connection that the first Western scientific work on botany was published in 1735 by a Swedish natural scientist and that it contained only 12 pages of classifications and appeared one-and-a-half centuries after *An Outline of Materia Medica*.

CHINESE MEDICINE IN MODERN TIMES

In the beginning of the twentieth century when Western medicine made its way into China along with other aspects of Western culture, the Chinese were greatly impressed by the apparently effective therapies of the West in curing many infectious and contagious diseases then widespread in China, such as malaria and cholera and other diseases that require surgery. By the year 1905, there were 166 hospitals and 241 clinics of Western medicine operated by Western physicians in China. The first college of Western medicine was established in Peking in 1906. By the year 1934, there was a total of 30 colleges of Western medicine in China, with 3,616 students enrolled and 532 graduates from them.

Due to this sudden impact of Western medicine, by 1914 many Chinese scholars had begun to advocate the abolition of traditional Chinese medicine. And in 1929 the Chinese government proposed legislation that would ban the practice of traditional Chinese medicine. However, the proposed legislation was not passed due to the strong opposition by the Chinese people in general and the Chinese physicians of traditional medicine in particular.

In 1930, the Chinese government passed legislation to separate Chinese medicine and Western medicine, and so, the first college of traditional Chinese medicine was established in China that same year. By this time, there were already over 400 journals of traditional Chinese medicine being published.

As time went on, most of the widespread diseases in China were gradually being brought under control, which allowed the Chinese people to pay greater attention to other less threatening but still equally important

16

chronic diseases, such as arthritis, heart disease, and diabetes. However, it didn't take long for the Chinese to realize the inadequacies of Western medicine in treating such diseases, and this realization caused them to reassess the value of traditional Chinese medicine. As a result of this reassessment, traditional Chinese medicine has gradually regained its proper place in the Chinese health care system.

In modern China, Chinese and Western medicine are practised side by side, and Chinese patients have the freedom to choose between the two, with both types equally available to them. In recent years, patterns reflecting their choices have emerged: Whenever their conditions obviously require surgery or when they are in a crisis situation, they will opt for Western medicine; but when they suffer from chronic diseases, such as rheumatism, hypertension, diabetes, and heart disease, they will choose Chinese medicine. It goes without saying, however, that the choice is not always an either-or proposition, and it's becoming a common practice for a Chinese patient to be treated by Chinese and Western medicine simultaneously, which is called the combined therapy of Chinese and Western medicine.

1
Classification of Chinese Herbs

The classification of various items under study marked the beginning of science, and has continued into modern times. In botany, for example, we classify plants into different families to further our understanding of them. Chinese herbs are as old as Chinese history, and the ancient Chinese classified herbs according to their basic actions—in other words, what they could do to the human body. There are a total of 20 major classifications within Chinese herbalism today, each of which represents a number of important actions.

1. CLASS OF HERBS TO INDUCE PERSPIRATION

The herbs that fall under this classification have one thing in common, namely, that they can induce perspiration, which is their major action. For this reason, an illness that can be alleviated by perspiration can be treated with this class of herbs. Conversely, a patient with an illness that can be intensified by perspiration should avoid this class of herbs. If, for example, you catch a cold, herbs in this class would benefit you, because in order to overcome the common cold or the flu, it is necessary to induce perspiration. On the other hand, if you suffer from night sweats, excessive perspiration, or chronic diarrhea, which will have already drained off a great deal of water from your body, you should avoid herbs in this class as much as possible.

Herbs that induce perspiration are divided into two subclasses: herbs for symptoms characterized by cold sensations (namely, Chinese ephedra, lily-flowered magnolia, and purple perilla) and herbs for symptoms characterized by fever (namely, hare's ear, kudzu vine, and mulberry-leaved chrysanthemum). Thus, if you are suffering from the common cold with chills, the first subclass of herbs should be used; but once you display high fever, the second subclass is recommended.

All classes of herbs have specific uses and also entail a few measures of

19

precaution. The major uses for the class of herbs that induce perspiration are the common cold and the flu as well as many related symptoms, such as headache, fever, pain in the body, and a cough. In addition, this class of herbs is also frequently used to treat bronchitis, bronchial asthma, measles at an early stage, acute glomerulonephritis, and acute rheumatic fever.

There are four measures of precaution in using this class of herbs. First, herbs in this class are not good for chronic symptoms involving the internal organs. This is partly because such symptoms cannot be treated simply by inducing perspiration, and partly because a prolonged consumption of these herbs will weaken the body, which is not desirable for patients suffering from chronic diseases of the internal organs. Second, symptoms that have already dehydrated the body, such as vomiting, diarrhea, and bleeding, should not be treated by this class of herbs. Third, after taking this class of herbs, it is desirable to stay calm and keep warm so that perspiration will occur to a suitable degree, being neither excessive nor insufficient. Fourth, when a rather weak patient such as an older person takes this class of herbs to heal an illness, it is wise for him or her to consume some herbs under the classification of herbs to treat deficiencies, namely, class 16.

From the point of view of modern medicine, the class of herbs to induce perspiration performs two basic functions. First, the herbs in this class can expand blood capillaries in the superficial region of the body and activate the secretion of the sweat gland in order to reduce fever, get rid of toxin, inhibit bacteria, and strengthen the body's ability to ingest and destroy bacteria and defend itself against foreign invasion. Second, this class of herbs can increase glomerular filtration to remove excessive water in the body.

2. CLASS OF HERBS TO REDUCE EXCESSIVE HEAT INSIDE THE BODY

Many diseases are due to the presence of excessive heat inside the body. This class of herbs is capable of reducing excessive heat inside the body, and is used for those diseases that are mostly characterized by inflammation or infection. This class is divided into three subclasses: herbs to reduce the "heat of fire" (namely, carrizo, cork tree, goldthread, purslane, self-heal, skullcap, and wind weed), herbs to reduce heat in the blood (namely, Chinese pulsatilla and white rose), and herbs to reduce heat and detoxicate at the same time (namely, Asian dandelion, chicken-bone grass, Chinese violet, Japanese honeysuckle, and puff ball).

The concept of heat is a unique concept in Chinese medicine, as heat is believed to be the cause of many so-called hot symptoms. Herbs that can reduce "heat of fire" are used to treat acute inflammatory and infectious diseases, because acute diseases can be said to attack as fast as fire burning

20

down a building. Such acute diseases include encephalitis, which is inflammation of the brain; pneumonia, which is inflammation of the lungs; and acute bronchitis, which is inflammation of the bronchial mucous membrane. Herbs that can reduce heat in the blood are used to arrest bleeding, such as with nosebleeds, discharge of blood from the mouth, and vaginal bleeding. Herbs that can reduce heat and detoxicate simultaneously are normally used to treat inflammatory and infectious diseases that are suppurative, such as many skin diseases, mumps, lymphangitis, mastitis, and appendicitis.

A few measures of precaution should be taken in using this class of herbs. First, symptoms related to the common cold or the flu and to fever or excessive heat in the body due to constipation should not be treated by this class of herbs. Second, herbs in this class tend to be bad for the stomach, because they are not easily digested; for this reason, they can be taken with the class of herbs for promoting digestion, if necessary (class 9). Third, this class of herbs can dehydrate the body, and for this reason, they can be taken with yin tonics, which consist of herbs to treat yin deficiency (class 16).

From the viewpoint of modern medicine, this class of herbs can be used to heal inflammation, counteract bacteria, arrest bleeding, reduce body temperature, increase urination, and activate the ureter, which explains why such herbs can treat urinary stones effectively.

3. CLASS OF HERBS TO COUNTERACT RHEUMATISM

Most of the herbs in this class can be used to relieve pain, and they are especially effective for the treatment of muscular pain and pain of arthritis and rheumatism. The herbs included under this classification are Chinese clematis, mistletoe, and slender acanthopanax root bark.

Arthritis and rheumatism, at the beginning stage, should be treated by herbs in this class along with those in the class to induce perspiration (class 1). As these illnesses enter the intermediate stage, they should be treated by this class of herbs along with the class of herbs to promote blood circulation (class 12).

The Chinese believe that rheumatism is caused by three factors, or any combination of them. These three factors are wind, cold, and dampness. When rheumatism is caused by wind, the pain travels around the entire body, which is why it is called wandering pain and is difficult for the patient to pinpoint. Chinese clematis and mistletoe are particularly good for arthritis and rheumatism caused by wind. When rheumatism is caused by dampness, the pain will stay in a fixed region, so that the patient can easily point to where the pain is occurring. Slender acanthopanax root bark is especially good for this type of rheumatism.

21

4. CLASS OF HERBS TO REDUCE COLD SENSATIONS INSIDE THE BODY

This class of herbs is used to warm the body in the treatment of ailments associated with cold sensations inside the body, such as vomiting, diarrhea, cold abdominal pain, cold stomachache, and poor appetite. Some people feel a need to vomit because of cold sensations in the stomach and others develop diarrhea due to cold sensations in the bowel. One herb in this class is called evodia; it is a warm herb and is frequently used to stop vomiting and relieve cold pain.

If you have a cold symptom such as vomiting or diarrhea, and you have also caught a cold and are not completely recovered, you can take this class of herbs along with the class of herbs to induce perspiration (class 1). As herbs that reduce cold sensations inside the body are warm and dry, they are not to be taken by people with a hot disease or by those whose water content in the body is in short supply.

From the standpoint of modern medicine, this class of herbs can improve the functions of the cardiovascular system, increase heart action, excite the vasomotor center and the sympathetic nervous system, elevate blood pressure, and improve blood circulation. In addition, these herbs have been found to improve the hypothalamo-hypophysial function and the function of the endocrine glands, as well as elevate the effects of the neurohumoral regulation for better coordination among various vital internal organs that will in turn improve metabolism.

5. CLASS OF HERBS TO REDUCE DAMPNESS IN THE BODY

When dampness accumulates in the body, it can cause many ailments, including abdominal swelling, swelling of the stomach, puffiness in the limbs, diarrhea, jaundice, and a few skin diseases. This class is divided into two subclasses: herbs to transform or absorb dampness (namely, buyuryo, grey atractylodes, and Korean mint) and herbs to promote urination (namely, Asiatic plantain, coin grass, and evergreen artemisia).

To transform dampness means to stimulate the action of the spleen so that it can speed up the excretion of water from the body. The Chinese believe that one reason why dampness continues to accumulate in the body is that the spleen is not strong enough to make water flow. The herbs that can transform dampness are able to correct the conditions of the spleen. Another way of getting rid of dampness inside the body is through promoting urination. The herbs for promoting urination are often used to treat many urination disturbances and related symptoms, such as edema, stones in the urinary system, and acute nephritis. In addition, many obese people have accumulated an excessive quantity of water in the body, which is why this class of herbs is often used for weight reduction.

Along with reducing dampness inside the body, this class of herbs, at the same time, can also reduce yin energy in the body. For this reason, people with dry conditions and thin and weak people should not use this class of herbs.

From the point of view of modern medicine, this class of herbs has been proven effective for cardiac-renal edema, nutritional edema, prostatomeg-aly urinary retention, and other symptoms associated with gastroenteric disturbances, such as nausea, vomiting, poor appetite, and diarrhea. These usages are attributed to the following three functions performed by this class of herbs: First, this class of herbs can enhance the functions of the heart, lungs, and kidneys; second, it can regulate the functions of the stomach and the intestines to stop many digestive disturbances; and third, it can adjust the neurohumoral regulation, which contributes to excretion of excessive water in the body.

6. CLASS OF HERBS FOR LUBRICATING DRY SYMPTOMS

A dry disease should be lubricated. Dry diseases can be either internal or external, and this class of herbs is used for treating both categories. Internal dryness may give rise to dry skin, constipation, discharge of dry and solid stools, discharge of scanty urine, thirst, dry throat with cracked lips, and sleeplessness; external dryness may give rise to absence of perspiration in hot weather, blood in sputum, dry cough, dry nose, and dry skin.

This class of herbs is divided into three subclasses. The first subclass consists of herbs for lubricating the lungs. Herbs in this subclass are used to treat dryness of the lungs and yin deficiency of the lungs, which can manifest in the following ailments: loss of voice, coughing up blood, dry cough, atrophic rhinitis, the common cold, influenza, bronchitis, diabetes insipidus, throat pain, dry nose and throat, and tickle in the throat. The second subclass consists of herbs for producing fluids and strengthening the stomach. These herbs are used to produce fluids in the stomach, mostly for the treatment of yin deficiency of the stomach, manifesting as diabetes mellitus, morbid hunger, dry lips, or stomachache. The third subclass consists of herbs for watering the yin (to increase yin energy in the body, as in watering a plant) and lubricating dryness of the intestines. These herbs are mostly used to treat yin exhaustion, dryness of the intestines, and dry constipation.

Herbs in this class can slow down movements inside the body, including energy circulation, blood circulation, and digestion. So, for this reason, those with poor energy circulation, poor blood circulation, or chronic in-digestion, should avoid this class of herbs.

23

7. CLASS OF HERBS TO INDUCE VOMITING

Most of the herbs in this class are very strong, which is why they can induce vomiting. Among them is the herb called black false hellebore, which is often used to induce vomiting of sputum and undigested foods, particularly in patients of epilepsy, apoplexy, thyroiditis, and lymphadenitis, in order to remove substances that may block the throat and obstruct breathing. Normally herbs in this class are available in powdered form.

If a patient fails to vomit within 10 to 20 minutes, he or she should use a finger to penetrate the throat to induce vomiting. If a patient continues to vomit without stop, some ginger juice, cold rice soup, or cold water can be administered to stop the vomiting. After vomiting, the patient should have some soup or semiliquid food and avoid greasy food and other food difficult to digest.

This class of herbs should not be consumed by patients with swallowing difficulty, asthma, a cough, pulmonary tuberculosis, aneurysm, arteriosclerosis, hypertension, or heart disease. Young and old patients, pregnant women, and weak patients should also avoid it.

8. CLASS OF HERBS TO INDUCE BOWEL MOVEMENTS

Herbs in this class, such as rhubarb, are most commonly used to treat constipation. However, many other diseases can also be treated by it, according to two treatment principles in Chinese medicine.

One treatment principle states that symptoms that occur in the upper region of the body can be treated by inducing bowel movements. Thus, inflammation of the eyes, ears, nose, mouth, and skin, and facial acne can be treated by this class of herbs as long as constipation or poor bowel movements are also indicated. The other treatment principle states that when smooth bowel movements are obstructed, abdominal pain and swelling may occur. These symptoms can be treated by this class of herbs so long as constipation or poor bowel movements are also indicated.

It's important to note that inducing bowel movements is a temporary measure in the treatment of an acute condition.

9. CLASS OF HERBS TO PROMOTE DIGESTION

This class of herbs is used to treat indigestion, swelling of the stomach, abdominal swelling, belching, nausea, vomiting, abdominal pain, diarrhea, and poor appetite. As a general rule, the symptoms to be treated by this class of herbs must be due to indigestion. Chinese hawthorn is an herb in this class.

Sometimes it may be necessary to use this class of herbs along with the class of herbs to regulate energy (class 11), because indigestion and poor

24

energy circulation are often associated with each other. When the herbs to promote digestion fail to work, it may be necessary to induce bowel movements as well, but both the herbs to promote digestion and the herbs to induce bowel movements (class 8) can only be used temporarily, as neither of them will contribute to the long-term health of the patient.

10. CLASS OF HERBS TO SUPPRESS COUGH AND REDUCE SPUTUM

This class of herbs can perform two actions simultaneously, namely, suppress coughing and reduce sputum. However, it is also frequently used to treat asthma, tuberculosis of the lymph node, goiter, epilepsy, and convulsions. This class of herbs is divided into three subclasses: First, herbs to reduce hot sputum (including antipyretic dichroa, snake gourd, and tendril-leaved fritillary bulb); second, herbs to suppress coughing and relieve asthma (including momordica fruit, sweet apricot, zuccarini's buttercup, and white cynanchum); and third, herbs to reduce cold sputum (such as jimson weed). Hot sputum appears yellowish whereas cold sputum appears white.

Herbs to reduce hot sputum are often used to treat tuberculosis of the lymph node and goiter; herbs to reduce cold sputum are often used to treat aching pain in the joints, as in arthritis; and herbs to suppress coughing and relieve asthma are often used to treat bronchitis, bronchial asthma, chronic cough, pulmonary tuberculosis, and tracheitis.

Since there are many different causes of sputum, the precise cause should be determined in order to treat it effectively. A cough with discharge of blood should not be treated by large dosages of herbs in this class in order to avoid additional bleeding. A cough associated with the common cold should be treated by this class of herbs along with the class of herbs to induce perspiration (class 1).

11. CLASS OF HERBS TO REGULATE ENERGY

Energy is a very fundamental concept in Chinese medicine, often compared with the blood. The energy in the body circulates the same way as blood circulates, and as with blood, energy can circulate too slowly, too quickly, or irregularly. When energy keeps flowing upwards, it can cause hiccups and vomiting; when it keeps flowing downwards, it can cause prolapse of the anus, the uterus, or the stomach. When energy flows too slowly, it can cause chest pain and depression. The class of herbs to regulate energy is used to make energy circulate smoothly in the body, and one such herb is yellow jasmine.

The ailments often treated by this class of herbs include chest pain, pain in the ribs, abdominal pain, vomiting, hiccups, prolapse of the anus, pro-

25

lapse of the uterus, prolapse of the stomach, menstrual pain, enteritis, and acute bronchitis.

However, herbs in this class travel very fast in the body, so they can use up a great deal of energy, not unlike a car that runs fast using up a great deal of gas and oil. For this reason, this class of herbs should not be used for a prolonged period of time.

The Chinese classify energy as yang and blood as yin. They are sister and brother, with energy as brother and blood as sister, and they travel in the body hand in hand. In order to ensure that they travel together smoothly, the herbs to regulate energy and the herbs to regulate blood (class 12) are often used together.

12. CLASS OF HERB TO REGULATE BLOOD

This class of herbs can regulate the blood in two different ways, which is why it is divided into two subclasses: first, herbs to promote blood circulation (including Siberian motherwort and two-toothed amaranthus) and second, herbs to arrest bleeding (including agrimony and pseudo-ginseng).

When the blood fails to circulate smoothly, one major result can be blood coagulation, which is responsible for many ailments. For example, blood coagulation can cause the suppression of menstruation, menstrual pain, abdominal pain after childbirth, and chest pain. External factors can also result in blood coagulation, such as injuries from an automobile accident, a fall from a high place, or lifting a heavy object in an improper manner. Some people experience pain in the chest, for example, long after an accident, which could be due to blood coagulation caused by the accident. Since blood coagulation occurs in many diseases, including thromboangiitis obliterans, coronary heart disease, and erythema nodosum, herbs in this class can be effective in their treatment. Herbs to arrest bleeding are used to treat bleeding of various kinds, including vomiting of blood, nosebleeds, discharge of blood from the anus, blood in the urine, vaginal bleeding, and bleeding from external causes.

13. CLASS OF HERBS TO REGAIN CONSCIOUSNESS

Sudden fainting often occurs in patients of apoplexy or epilepsy, and with those suffering from convulsions or high fever. In apoplexy, for example, in order to arouse a patient who has fainted, it may be necessary to administer the herb by hand, which is one reason why this class of herbs comes in tablets and powder.

There are two different ways of suffering from loss of consciousness; one is called the "closed type" and the other is called the "prolapse type," and each should be treated differently. When a patient faints with closed fists, a locked jaw, rough breathing, and a strong pulse, it is a closed type and

26

should be treated by herbs in this class, such as benzoin. But when a patient faints with open hands, a pale complexion, and a weak pulse, it is a prolapse type, which should be treated by ginseng, an herb in class 16.

14. CLASS OF HERBS TO REDUCE ANXIETY

This class of herbs is often used to treat insomnia, excessive dreaming, forgetfulness, palpitations, epilepsy, convulsions, dizziness, depression, night sweats, excessive perspiration, and a congested chest. Oriental arborvitae seed belongs to this class of herbs. However, when these ailments are due to blood deficiency, they should be treated by this class of herbs along with the class of herbs to treat blood deficiency, also referred to as blood tonics (class 16).

15. CLASS OF HERBS TO STOP INVOLUNTARY MOVEMENTS

Involuntary movements are often manifested as a shaking of the head or of the hands, or muscular twitching, as observed in apoplexy. Tuber of elevated gastrodia belongs to this class of herbs. Herbs in this class are often used along with herbs in other classes, because frequently patients with involuntary movement problems also display other symptoms as well. For example, when a patient also suffers from insomnia and palpitations, the class of herbs to reduce anxiety (class 14) should be used in combination.

16. CLASS OF HERBS TO CORRECT DEFICIENCIES

This class of herbs plays a fundamental role in Chinese medicine, and its major function is to make the body stronger. In the terminology of Western medicine, this class of herbs could be called the class of herbs to enhance the body's immune function, but there is a basic difference between the Chinese and the Western approaches in this connection. Western scientists believe that if something can enhance the body's immune function, it must be good for everybody, but it is maintained in Chinese medicine that the body can be strengthened only in accordance with the nature of its weaknesses. A person may be strong in certain respects and weak in others, and it is essential to determine exactly what the weak aspects are of each individual before this class of herbs can be used effectively.

In Chinese medicine, when a person has a weakness, it is called a "deficiency." There are four types of deficiencies: energy deficiency, which means low energy; yang deficiency, which means weak kidneys in general and low sexual capacity in particular; blood deficiency, which means either shortage or poor quality of blood; and yin deficiency, which means shortage of body fluids.

27

This class of herbs is divided into four subclasses based on the four types of deficiency. The first subclass consists of herbs to treat energy deficiency, and they are called energy tonics. Chinese ginseng, Chinese yam, licorice, membraneous milk vetch, and red date, belong to this subclass. The second subclass consists of herbs to treat yang deficiency, which are called yang tonics, and dodder, eucommia bark, longspur epimedium, morinda root, snake-bed seed, snow lotus, and teasel belong to this subclass. The third subclass consists of herbs to treat blood deficiency, which are called blood tonics, and danggui, glutinous rehmannia, and tuber of multiflower knotweed belong to it. And the fourth subclass consists of herbs to treat yin deficiency, which are called yin tonics; lily, matrimony vine, sealwort, sesame, tremella, wax tree, and white peony belong to it.

Herbs for treating energy deficiency are effective for shortness of breath, asthma, fatigue, low body weight, poor appetite, indigestion, diarrhea, abdominal swelling, puffiness, prolapse of the uterus and the anus, and prolapse of the stomach. Herbs for treating yang deficiency are effective for lumbago, cold limbs, frequent urination, impotence, seminal emission, chronic diarrhea, abdominal pain, infertility, and blurred vision. Herbs for treating blood deficiency are effective for palpitations, forgetfulness, insomnia, headaches, dizziness, ringing in the ears, irregular menstruation, muscular twitching, opisthotonos, night sweats, and diabetes. Herbs for treating yin deficiency are effective for a chronic cough, night sweats, seminal emission, hoarseness, constant thirst, a chronic sore throat, a dry cough, excessive perspiration, lumbago, blurred vision, ringing in the ears, and diabetes.

According to a report published in 1983 by the Chinese Academy of Medical Science, this class of herbs can be effectively used in the treatment of chronic tracheitis, atherosclerosis, coronary heart disease, glomerulonephritis, hyperthyroidism, chronic atrophic gastritis, hepatitis B, rheumatoid arthritis, lupus erythematosus, scleroderma, pulseless disease, Behcet's disease, tumors, organic transplantation, and aging, as well as in the prevention of the common cold.

17. CLASS OF HERBS TO CONSTRICT AND OBSTRUCT MOVEMENTS

To constrict means to tighten up, thus making movements more difficult, and to obstruct means to slow down the movements by making the passage rougher. This class of herbs is divided into two subclasses. The first subclass consists of herbs that can constrict and obstruct the movement of semen in men, and of urination (such as cherokee rose). The second subclass consists of herbs that can constrict and obstruct bowel movements (such as water lily). Herbs that can constrict and obstruct the movement of semen in men, and of urination, are used to treat premature ejaculation during sexual intercourse, seminal emission, enuresis, and frequent urination. Herbs that can constrict and obstruct bowel movements are mostly used to check diarrhea.

However, this class of herbs is only used to deal with these problems symptomatically, which means that it cannot be used as a fundamental cure. For instance, when diarrhea occurs, this class of herbs should be used only when the real cause of it cannot be identified; otherwise, the herbal treatment should be directed towards the cause. If the diarrhea is caused by indigestion, it should be treated by the class of herbs that promote digestion (class 9); if it is caused by cold sensations in the bowel, it should be treated by the class of herbs that warm the body (class 4).

18. CLASS OF HERBS TO EXPEL OR DESTROY PARASITES

Parasites can cause intermittent abdominal pain, vomiting of bubbles, grinding of teeth at night, poor appetite, morbid hunger, love of strange foods, itch in the anus or the ears or the nose, a withered and yellowish complexion, and puffiness all over the body. Such problems should be treated by this class of herbs according to the types of parasites involved.

The herbs to expel or destroy parasites should be administered on an empty stomach, so that they will produce stronger effects on the parasites. The patient taking such herbs should rest well and avoid greasy foods, and after the parasites have been expelled, should take some tonics (class 16) to facilitate early recovery.

This class of herbs should not be administered to pregnant women, young or weak patients, and patients with high fever or acute abdominal pain.

19. CLASS OF HERBS FOR ULCERS AND TUMORS

The Chinese have developed three basic strategies against ulcers and tumors. The first strategy is to boost the patient's immune system, particularly if the patient is weak or old, so that the body can fight off the disease. The second strategy is to attack the ulcers and tumors by clearing toxic heat in the body. And the third strategy is to make certain that blood and energy are circulating properly.

The herbs to boost the immune system are presented under class 16, the herbs to promote blood circulation are presented under class 11, and the herbs to promote energy circulation are presented under class 12. The herbs that attack ulcers and tumors by clearing toxic heat are in this class, and are fairly strong herbs that should be used with great care.

This class of herbs is divided into six subclasses. The first subclass consists of herbs for reducing heat, counteracting toxic effects, and healing

29

swelling. The second subclass consists of herbs for reducing heat, benefitting water metabolism, and removing dampness. The third consists of herbs for removing sputum and dispersing coagulations. The fourth consists of herbs for transforming sputum and softening up hardness. The fifth consists of herbs for opening up the passages of meridians and activating them. And the sixth consists of other miscellaneous herbs for ulcers and tumors.

20. CLASS OF HERBS FOR EXTERNAL APPLICATIONS

Herbs in this class are used for boils, carbuncles, fractures, and bleeding due to external injuries. Such herbs can counteract toxic effects, heal swelling, remove pus, and relieve pain. Although some of these herbs can also be consumed internally, most of them are toxic and should be taken with caution.

This class of herbs is divided into six subclasses. The first subclass consists of herbs for destroying worms and counteracting toxic effects. The second consists of herbs for healing swelling, dispersing coagulations, and softening up hardness. The third consists of herbs for expelling pus and transforming decay. The fourth consists of herbs for activating the blood and removing wind (for more about the ill effects of wind, turn to pages 31–35). The fifth consists of herbs for the arrestment of bleeding through constrictive effects. And the sixth is made up of other miscellaneous herbs for external application.

2

The Chinese View of the Causes of Disease

What causes disease? In Western medicine, germs and viruses are the primary culprits. But in Chinese medicine, the causes of disease are divided into three basic categories: first, external causes, which include six atmospheric energies (namely, wind, cold, summer heat, dampness, dryness, and fire); second, internal causes, which include seven emotions (namely, joy, anger, worry, thought, sadness, fear, and shock); and third, two other causes that are neither internal nor external, fatigue and foods. How do we know that such factors cause disease? Our knowledge of them has not come from laboratory research but rather from common experience. For instance, we know from experience that we will get sick when we are constantly exposed to wind or cold or summer heat, or when we are extremely fatigued or when we constantly overeat.

These causes of disease are very familiar to all of us, even though many of us may not pay much attention to them. A mother, for example, will seldom, if ever, ask a child with a bad cold where or when he got the virus, but rather when he forgot to put on warm clothes or whether he kept himself warm in bed the night before. We cannot see germs or viruses with the naked eye, but we do know that under certain circumstances we are more likely to get sick, and this knowledge is based on common experience. Since traditional Chinese medicine has grown out of common human experience of over 2,000 years, germs and viruses are seen to play no part in the causes of disease; instead, the main focus is on the other factors familiar in common experience.

WIND

How does the wind cause disease? Wind is a natural phenomenon in the atmosphere; it is air in motion, and we need it to maintain good health. When we feel hot, for example, we need wind to cool us down, and we leave our windows open on purpose in the summer, because we need fresh air that the wind will blow in. Therefore, as a natural atmospheric

31

energy, wind is essential to human health; but, depending on the circumstances, wind, like anything else, can be either beneficial or harmful to our health. When wind causes disease, it obviously becomes harmful to the human body, and in Chinese medicine, when this happens, wind is regarded as a hostile atmospheric energy to be avoided.

The six atmospheric energies are called hostile energies when they cause disease, and they are in opposition to the energy in the body, which is called body energy. Hence, in Chinese medicine, disease is the result of a struggle between hostile energies and body energy, not unlike the struggle between germs or viruses and the immune system in Western medicine.

How do we know that a specific disease is caused by the wind? Over the years, Chinese physicians have analyzed the nature of wind very carefully, and they have found various distinct characteristics of the wind to be linked with certain symptoms and diseases.

Wind is the dominant atmospheric energy in spring, but it occurs in all seasons. There is warm wind in spring, hot and damp wind in summer, cool and dry wind in autumn, and cold wind in winter. Since wind occurs virtually in all seasons, it is a friend of other atmospheric energies, and, as such, it can team up with them to cause disease. For example, wind and cold often team up to cause the common cold and the flu, and such ailments are called "wind cold" in Chinese. Wind and dampness often team up to cause arthritis and rheumatism, and such illnesses are called "wind dampness." And wind and dryness often team up to cause a dry cough and a dry throat, which are called "wind dryness." Since the wind occurs in all seasons and can team up with other hostile energies to cause disease, the Chinese maintain that the wind is the foremost cause of disease. There are three specific circumstances under which people are most susceptible to the attack of wind: when they are exposed to the wind while perspiring, just getting up from bed, or right after taking a bath.

Wind is a yang hostile energy. It is the nature of yang to move upwards and stay high; so, if you want to avoid wind on stormy days, you should stay as low as possible. The wind often attacks the upper region of the body, causing such symptoms as a headache, sore throat, or cough, which are all common symptoms of a bad cold. When wind attacks the head causing a headache, it is called "head wind" in Chinese. There is a type of edema that involves the head and the face, and especially the area below the eyes, which is called "kidney wind," because it's due to the wind attacking the kidneys. Severe edema in the upper part of the body is called "wind water," because it's caused by wind carrying water that invades the upper body. A type of disease called erysipelas that is characterized by inflammation and swelling of the face with difficulty in opening one's eyes is called "greater head wind," because it's caused by a major attack of the wind. A skin disease known as vitiligo that is characterized by white patches on the head is called "white patches wind," because it's caused by the simultaneous attack of wind and dampness.

Since the wind is a leading cause of the common cold, people suffering from the common cold or the flu often have nasal congestion and a cough, which are symptoms involving the upper part of the body. Facial paralysis is another common symptom caused by the wind, because the face is seldom covered, which makes it frequently exposed to the wind, and because the face is located in the upper region, making it most susceptible to the attack of the wind.

The nature of the wind is such that it moves fast and constantly undergoes rapid change. When a patient is under an attack of the wind, the symptoms often move from one place to another and also undergo rapid change, but they seldom last very long. For example, there is a type of rheumatism characterized by wandering pain that is caused by the wind. This wandering pain bears a close resemblance to the nature of wind in that it moves from one place to another without residing in one fixed spot. This type of rheumatism is called "wind rheumatism" in Chinese. When the wind attacks the joints causing a type of arthritis that affects the joints virtually all over the body, not necessarily simultaneously, it is called "joints swept by wind." Another distinct example is a type of skin itch that can occur in any part of the body, just like wind that moves from one place to another; it is called "wind itch."

Since wind is air in motion, when it attacks the body, it often causes shaking symptoms, not unlike a tree shaken by strong winds. When we see someone suffering from dizziness in the head with a twirling sensation, from shaking of the arms and legs, or from muscular twitching, the person is most likely under an attack of the wind. Tetanus is a disease characterized by stiffness and spasm of the muscles and lockjaw, and it is called "wind intruding into the wound" in Chinese. When people with epilepsy have a seizure, they often give a shrill cry and fall unconscious. The Chinese call this "goat wind" because it is caused by an attack of the wind and the cry is similar to that of a goat. And during the summer, when a person develops high fever, a desire to sleep, plus muscular spasm and twitching, this constellation of symptoms is called "summer wind," because it's caused by a simultaneous attack of wind and summer heat.

As with all atmospheric energies, when the wind attacks the body, it starts with the skin and then gradually moves inside the body. When wind causes the common cold, it is normally not a serious illness, but if the person takes it lightly and fails to treat it, the wind may continue to penetrate into the body to cause pneumonia with serious consequences.

There are five major internal organs and each of them is particularly susceptible to the attack of one specific atmospheric energy. The liver is most susceptible to the attack of wind, the kidneys are most susceptible to the attack of cold, the heart is most susceptible to the attack of summer heat, the spleen is most susceptible to the attack of dampness, and the lungs are most susceptible to the attack of dryness. All the organs are equally susceptible to the attack of fire.

When wind attacks the liver, it normally does not cause inflammation of the liver, known as hepatitis, nor does it cause jaundice, which is also a form of liver disease. After wind has penetrated into the internal region of the body, it is no longer an external hostile energy but an internal one. As wind attacks the liver, the liver starts to shake, and although we do not see it shake, we can observe the victim suffering from shaking symptoms, such as shaking of the head and hands, twitching of muscles, wry eye or wry mouth, and sudden fainting. In Chinese medicine, the liver is compared to a tree, with the head, limbs, eyes, mouth, and muscles viewed as its leaves and branches. The Chinese refer to the shaking symptoms as the symptoms of "liver wind." Such symptoms develop when the liver is under the attack of internal wind.

How do we treat diseases caused by the wind with herbs? Wind can attack the body at three different levels: the superficial level, the medial level, and the deep level. Each of these levels involves different sets of symptoms that should be treated differently.

When wind attacks at the superficial level, a few of the following symptoms may occur: fear of wind, perspiration, nasal congestion and discharge, itch in the throat, a cough, a headache, fever at a later stage, and skin rash. Among the many diseases caused by wind attacking at the superficial level are these common ones in Western medicine: infections of the upper respiratory system and urticaria, which is a skin disease characterized by the eruption of pale evanescent wheals with severe itching. Symptoms and diseases such as these should be treated by the class of herbs to induce perspiration (class 1).

When wind attacks at the medial level, a few of the following symptoms may occur: wandering pain in the joints and limbs, acute stiffness of the joints and limbs, stiff neck, wry mouth and eyes, numbness of facial skin and muscles, twitching of the arms and legs, and lockjaw. Among the many diseases caused by wind attacking at the medial level are the following three common diseases in Western medicine: rheumatic arthritis, facial paralysis, and tetanus or lockjaw. Such symptoms and diseases should be treated by the class of herbs to counteract rheumatism (class 3) and the class of herbs to stop involuntary movements (class 15).

When wind attacks at the deep level, it is called "liver wind," as previously mentioned, and a few of the following symptoms can occur: headache, dizziness, wry mouth and eyes, numbness of the limbs, shaking of the head or hands, stiff tongue or the tongue slanting to one side, unclear speech or speech difficulty, and sudden fainting. Two disorders in Western medicine—hypertension and stroke or apoplexy—are among the many disorders and diseases caused by "liver wind." Such symptoms and diseases should be treated by the class of herbs to stop involuntary movements (class 15), the class of herbs to correct deficiencies (class 16), and the class of herbs to regulate the blood (class 12). The Chinese believe that in order to counteract "liver wind," it is necessary to tone the blood and

34

promote blood circulation. A common phrase in Chinese medicine to describe this strategy is "When the blood begins to circulate, wind will stop by itself." Blood deficiency is an important factor in the attack of "liver wind"; therefore, once external wind has become "liver wind," it is important to tone the blood and promote its circulation.

COLD

Cold is the dominant atmospheric energy in winter. When the body is under the attack of the cold, the person will experience dislike of the cold, fever, absence of perspiration, headaches, and pain in the body. When the cold attacks the digestive system, it will cause intestinal rumbling, diarrhea, and abdominal pain. The kidneys are most susceptible to the attack of cold, and when they are under attack, the person most often develops lower-back pain, cold feet, cold sensations in the genitals, and impotence.

Cold is most harmful to yang energy. Yang energy circulates in the superficial region to protect the body, not unlike soldiers defending a country against foreign invasion; yin energy, on the other hand, is situated in the deeper region to nourish the internal organs. When cold attacks the body, the first victim is yang energy. When yang energy is under the attack of the cold, shivering sensations are caused at first, but gradually the pores are blocked up by the invading cold energy so that the person becomes unable to perspire. After the cold has defeated the yang energy and has victoriously penetrated into the body, the pores become almost completely shut off due to the cold, so that body heat has nowhere to go and thus accumulates inside the body. The accumulated body heat is finally forced to break open the blocked pores, which is why the person begins to perspire profusely at this juncture.

The nature of the cold is to contract or to freeze, so to speak. Perniosis, or chilblain, is a skin disorder caused by the cold, and the Chinese call it "frozen injury." Frostbite is characterized by the freezing of a part or parts of the body, particularly the nose, the fingers, and the toes, and the Chinese call it "frozen carbuncle." When cold attacks the surface of the skin, it causes absence of perspiration, and skin numbness, and it makes one's hair stand on end; when it attacks the tendons and bones, it causes shivering, spasms, and rheumatism; and when it attacks the joints, it causes arthritis. All these symptoms are due to the nature of cold—namely, cold freezes skin, muscles, bones, and joints. Since cold causes pain by freezing the affected part, the pain always stays in the same spot and appears very severe. Thus, rheumatism caused by cold is called "painful rheumatism" in Chinese. Also, hernias of various sorts are caused by cold, and for that reason, are called "cold hernias" in Chinese.

Cold is clear in nature, and as such, it often causes clear symptoms. For example, clear nasal discharge, a symptom of the common cold, is due to wind and cold teaming up to attack the nose, and is called "wind cold" in

Chinese. Coughing up clear mucus is due to cold attacking the lungs, and is called "cold lungs" in Chinese. Vomiting of clear water is due to cold attacking the stomach, which is called "cold stomach." Discharge of clear urine, as in frequent urination, and discharge of clear stools, as in diarrhea, are both due to the attack of cold while the body is in a weak state.

When the cold penetrates deep into the internal region to cause disease, it becomes an internal hostile energy and is called internal cold. Internal cold reduces body heat so that a person will have cold limbs and a pale complexion, and will experience shivering, nausea, vomiting, diarrhea, and abdominal rumbling and pain, as well as loss of consciousness in severe cases. When a disease is caused by cold, the patient will feel relieved by warmness, such as eating hot foods or exposure to heat. Internal cold can also be caused by other factors, including frequent consumption of foods with cold energy and loss of internal heat for various reasons but mostly those associated with a hypofunctioning of the body.

The Chinese traditionally divide internal cold into two categories: middle cold and lower cold. Middle cold refers to the attack of the middle part of the abdominal cavity by cold energy, which often gives rise to vomiting of clear water, cold arms and legs, and a pale complexion. Lower cold refers to the attack of the lower part of the abdominal cavity by cold energy, often causing discharge of long streams of clear urine, diarrhea, impotence, cold arms and legs, and fatigue.

How do we use herbs in dealing with the attack of the cold? This depends on the mode of attack—whether the cold attacks at the superficial level, at the deep region, or at the internal region, threatening the patient's life.

When the cold only attacks at the superficial level, some of the following ailments may occur: dislike of the cold, fever without perspiration, headache with a stiff neck, pain in the body, asthma with coughing, pain in the bones, severe pain in a fixed region that can be relieved by warmness but intensified by cold, and difficulty in moving the affected parts. Quite a few diseases in Western medicine are caused by cold attacking at the superficial level, such as the common cold, the flu, and arthritis. Other diseases in Western medicine frequently triggered by cold at this level are bronchial asthma, fibrositis (inflammation of the fibrous connective tissues), and bursitis (inflammation of a cavity in the vicinity of joints). These types of ailments should be treated by the class of herbs to counteract rheumatism (class 3), to reduce cold sensations inside the body (class 4), and to induce perspiration (class 1).

When cold attacks the deep region, it is an internal cold affecting the kidneys and the spleen in particular. In such cases, a few of the following symptoms may occur: pale complexion, fatigue, cold sensations (particularly in the arms and legs) that can be relieved by heat, diarrhea in the early morning, abdominal pain, puffiness in the lower arms and legs, and ascites (accumulation of fluids in the peritoneal cavity). Among the many diseases

36

in Western medicine caused by internal cold are chronic inflammation of the intestine (chronic enteritis), intestinal tuberculosis, chronic inflammation of the kidneys (chronic nephritis), and cirrhotic ascites (accumulation of fluids in the peritoneal cavity in liver disease). These types of symptoms and diseases should be treated by the class of herbs to correct deficiencies (class 16) and the class of herbs to reduce cold sensations inside the body (class 4).

When cold penetrates into the body, directly attacking the internal region and threatening the life of the patient, a few of the following symptoms may occur: shivering with cold, numbness of the arms and legs, the limbs feeling as cold as ice, spasmodic cold pain, clenching teeth, loss of consciousness with the body becoming cold and stiff, slow and feeble breathing, cold air coming from the mouth and nose, and the skin turning purple. These types of symptoms should be treated by the class of herbs to reduce cold sensations inside the body (class 4).

SUMMER HEAT

Summer heat is the dominant atmospheric energy in early and middle summer, when people often experience high fever, thirst, and profuse perspiration, all of which are hot symptoms. But, more importantly, summer heat is especially harmful to body fluids, as it is the nature of summer heat to suck moisture and water from the body. This explains why a person under the attack of summer heat will feel extremely thirsty and very fatigued due to a lack of body fluids, and will have a dry mouth and lips, constipation due to dry intestines, and scanty urine due to a shortage of water in the body. Among the internal organs, the heart is most susceptible to the attack of summer heat. When summer heat attacks the heart, it may cause eye infection, thirst, nosebleeds, and vomiting of blood, as well as a loss of consciousness in severe cases.

Summer heat and dampness often team up to attack the body. This is not only because summer heat is the dominant atmospheric energy in the summer, and there is high humidity in the summer, but because people also tend to consume more water and beverages in the summer. When the two hostile energies attack the body simultaneously, the most distinct symptoms are a congested chest, nausea with a desire to vomit, and poor appetite. Also, an attack of summer heat and dampness often cause one to feel thirsty but with no desire to drink.

An attack of summer heat may be either light or severe. When the attack is light, the symptoms are fever, thirst, perspiration, headache, nausea, vomiting, diarrhea, discharge of short streams of red urine, fatigue, shortness of breath, and a fatigued feeling in the arms and legs. When the attack is severe, it is called sunstroke, and the symptoms are extreme prostration, high fever, a red face, either no perspiration or perspiration with cold sweats, delirium, and collapse.

The Chinese also draw a distinction between yin summer heat and yang summer heat, with two distinct sets of symptoms. Yin summer heat refers to the attack of cold during hot summer, which occurs when people feel hot and try to counteract it by exposing themselves to cold wind or cold water or by consuming cold foods in large amounts. This type of attack is called the attack by yin summer heat, because the attacking energy is in fact cold, which is yin, and the attack takes place during the height of summer heat. Common symptoms of yin summer heat are fear of the cold, fever, no perspiration, heavy sensations in the body with pain, fatigue, vomiting, diarrhea, and a congested chest. Yang summer heat, on the other hand, refers to the attack of summer heat during the hot summer, which occurs when a person works long hours or takes a long journey under the hot sun. This type of attack is called the attack of yang summer heat, because the person under attack is on the move, which is yang in nature, and the attack takes place during the height of summer heat, which is also yang in nature. Hence, this type of attack can be viewed as two yang energies on a collision course. The most common symptoms of yang summer heat are stress, constant thirst, difficult urination, headaches, and hot sensations through-out the body. Both light and severe cases of summer heat, as mentioned earlier, fall under this yang summer heat category.

How can herbs be used to treat an attack of summer heat? There are three different modes of attack by summer heat—one at the superficial level, one that causes sunstroke, and one that is teamed up with dampness—and each should be treated by different herbs.

When summer heat attacks at the superficial level of the body, a few of the following symptoms may occur: headache with dizziness, head swelling, congested chest, nausea or vomiting, hot sensations in the body, thirst, fatigued limbs, dry skin with redness and hot sensations, scanty perspiration or profuse perspiration with cold skin, discharge of short streams of yellowish urine, and dry tongue. These types of symptoms should be treated by the class of herbs to reduce excessive heat inside the body (class 2) and the class of herbs for lubricating dry symptoms (class 6).

When summer heat causes sunstroke, a few of the following symptoms may occur: high fever, profuse perspiration or no perspiration, thirst, jumpiness, muscular twitching, palpitations, fainting, extreme prostration, delirium, collapse, and unclear thinking. Such symptoms should be treated by the class of herbs to reduce excessive heat inside the body (class 2) and the class of herbs for lubricating dry symptoms (class 6).

When summer heat teams up with dampness to attack the body, in addition to the symptoms mentioned earlier, it causes a number of diseases in Western medicine, such as viral infections, inflammation of the stomach (gastritis), and inflammation of the intestine (enteritis) in the summer. Such diseases should be treated by the class of herbs to reduce excessive heat inside the body (class 2) and the class of herbs to reduce dampness in the body (class 5).

38

DAMPNESS

Dampness is the dominant atmospheric energy in late summer, when summer rains make the ground very damp and the cooler weather prevents it from drying as quickly as it does earlier in the summer. When people walk in the rain, sleep on damp ground, live in a damp environment, wear wet clothes, or swim a lot, they become an easy target for an attack of dampness. Any symptom with a trait of water is caused by dampness, such as skin blisters, retention of water with puffiness, and diarrhea with watery stools.

A skin disease known as eczema that is characterized by papular lesions with suppuration is called "damp rash" in Chinese, because it is primarily caused by dampness invading the skin. Coughing up watery mucus that makes a noise in the throat, with chest congestion and panting, is called "damp phlegm obstructing the lungs." Vomiting of clear water, with the sound of water in the intestine, is called "stoppage of dampness in the middle region"; puffiness all over the body, with retention of water throughout the body and difficult urination, is called "flooding of dampness"; and rheumatism and arthritis, with pain that always stays in the same spot, is called "damp rheumatism" or "damp arthritis." Dampness tends to attack the joints, because it easily flows into the joints like water. Patients with rheumatism, arthritis, and osteoarthritis (a degenerative joint disease) caused by dampness often experience a worsening of symptoms when humidity is high.

Dampness is muddy and moves slowly, as opposed to cold, which is clear in nature and moves more freely. Because of its slow movement, dampness often causes diseases that take a long time to heal; in this respect, dampness is the opposite of wind, which moves fast. When dampness causes pain as in rheumatism and arthritis, the pain always stays in the same spot, and as time goes on, swelling will occur due to an accumulation of dampness in the affected region. When dampness causes headaches, one feels dull pain in the head and sleepy and as if one's head were wrapped in a wet towel.

Dampness is heavy, with a tendency to move downwards to attack the lower part of the body, as opposed to wind, which is light, with a tendency to move upwards to attack the upper body. Since dampness tends to attack the lower body, a person under such an attack often displays swelling of the legs, feels that the legs are too heavy for walking, and has a sense of the entire body sinking down. Dampness and heat often work together to cause all sorts of symptoms, including discharge of yellowish urine, frequent but difficult urination, and vaginal discharge with an offensive smell in women. These symptoms are called "symptoms of damp heat" in Chinese medicine.

As with other atmospheric energies, when dampness attacks the body, it begins with the skin and then gradually penetrates into the body to become an internal hostile energy. Among the internal organs, the spleen is most susceptible to the attack of dampness. When dampness attacks the spleen, it is called "damp spleen," and the person may experience heavy sensations in the body, edema, a congested chest, poor appetite, and chronic diarrhea, and feel too lazy to even talk. When a person has nausea with a desire to vomit, a congested chest, abdominal swelling, poor appetite, indigestion, diarrhea with discharge of watery stools, and a light or sweet taste in the mouth, his or her stomach is under the attack of internal dampness. When dampness attacks the intestine, it causes diarrhea with a discharge of watery stools, which is understandable since dampness is a type of water.

As dampness has a natural tendency to attack the lower part of the body, it often causes rheumatism and arthritis in the legs, eczema in the legs, and wet beriberi, which is a vitamin B_1 deficiency disease characterized by swollen legs and feet, as well as by numbness, walking difficulty, difficult urination, and cold arms and legs.

How do we use herbs in treating an attack of dampness? There are four different modes of attack by dampness—one at the superficial level, one at the medial level, one of the skin, and one that penetrates into the internal regions. Each of these modes require different herbal cures.

When dampness attacks at the superficial level, a few of the following symptoms may occur: low fever over a prolonged period, slight fear of the cold, sticky sweats, heavy sensations in the head, pain in the arms and legs, congested chest, discharge of watery stools, discharge of abundant urine, and sticky sensations in the mouth without thirst. Viral infections, salmonella infection, and early stages of typhoid fever are among the diseases in Western medicine caused by this mode of attack. Such symptoms and diseases should be treated by the class of herbs to induce perspiration (class 1), to reduce excessive heat inside the body (class 2), and to reduce dampness in the body (class 5).

When dampness attacks at the medial level, some of these symptoms may occur: pain in the limbs and joints in a fixed region, swelling of the legs and knees and joints, difficulty in turning the body around, and puffiness in the legs. Rheumatic arthritis is a disease in Western medicine caused by dampness attacking at the medial level. Disorders such as these should be treated by the class of herbs to counteract rheumatism (class 3) and the class to reduce dampness in the body (class 5).

When dampness attacks the skin, it is called "toxic dampness soaking the skin," and a few of the following ailments may occur: scabies, painful and itchy skin blisters, and skin diseases characterized by the presence of pus. Many skin diseases in Western medicine are caused by toxic dampness soaking the skin, such as eczema, herpes simplex, impetigo (skin inflammation with isolated pustules), and tinea in the hands and feet. Such disorders should be treated by the class of herbs to reduce excessive heat

40

inside the body (class 2) as well as the class of herbs to reduce dampness in the body (class 5).

Finally, when dampness penetrates into the internal regions, attacking the spleen and stomach in particular, a few of the following symptoms may occur: a feeling of fullness in the stomach with poor appetite, abdominal swelling, discharge of soft stools, scanty urine, swollen feet, and sticky sensations in the mouth. Edema and bronchial asthma are two common diseases in Western medicine caused by internal dampness. These types of symptoms and diseases should be treated by the class of herbs to reduce excessive heat inside the body (class 2), to reduce dampness in the body (class 5), and to correct deficiencies (class 16).

DRYNESS

Dryness is the dominant energy in autumn, when there is low humidity in the atmosphere. Therefore, people are more susceptible to the attack of dryness at this time of year, and often experience such symptoms as dry cough, sore throat with dryness, dry skin, dry nose, thirst, scanty urine, and constipation with dry stools. An attack causing such symptoms is called "autumn dryness" in Chinese medicine.

Unlike other hostile atmospheric energies that attack the body through the skin and muscles, dryness attacks the body through the nose and mouth. For that reason, it can directly affect the lungs; so, among the internal organs, the lungs are most susceptible to the attack of dryness. One reason why smoking is particularly harmful to the lungs is that it makes them dry.

When dryness attacks the body in early autumn, it often teams up with the mild heat left over from the summer. This combined attack is called "warm dryness" in Chinese medicine. The symptoms include low fever, perspiration, thirst, sore throat, cough, pain in the ribs, dry nose, coughing up phlegm containing blood, and discharge of short streams of yellowish urine. On the other hand, when dryness attacks the body in late autumn, it often teams up with coolness, and is called "cool dryness." The symptoms include headache, dislike of the cold, dry coughs, no perspiration, nasal congestion, and a tickle in the throat.

Internal dryness mostly originates from the internal conditions of the body itself, so the Chinese refer to this kind of attack as an "internal production of dryness." It is mostly associated with excessive consumption of alcohol and spices, excessive perspiration, vomiting, chronic diarrhea, excessive bleeding, and chronic illnesses, all of which take a heavy toll on body fluids. Internal dryness causes dry skin, withered and broken hair, night sweats, morbid hunger, constipation with dry stools, discharge of scanty urine, hot sensations in the nostrils, poor vision, dry throat with cracked lips, sleeplessness, as well as light and periodic fever.

How do we treat dryness with herbs? As with the other atmospheric energies, the herbal treatments depend on the modes of attack. Dryness can attack at the superficial level; it can attack the lungs; and it can be internal.

When dryness attacks at the superficial level, some of the following symptoms may occur: dry skin, dry lips, dry mouth, dry nose, dry cough, and dry throat. Such symptoms should be treated by the class of herbs to reduce excessive heat inside the body (class 2) and the class for lubricating dry symptoms (class 6).

When dryness attacks the lungs, it can cause a dry cough, panting, a dry nose and throat, thirst, loss of voice, coughing up blood, presence of sputum that cannot be coughed up easily, and a sore throat. A few diseases in Western medicine that are caused by dryness attacking the lungs are atrophic rhinitis (chronic inflammation of the nasal mucosa, characterized by dry throat and hoarseness), bronchitis, and diabetes characterized by thirst. Such symptoms and diseases should be treated by the class of herbs for lubricating dry symptoms (class 6) and the class for suppressing cough and reducing sputum (class 10).

The symptoms associated with internal dryness have already been discussed. To treat these symptoms, use the class of herbs to reduce excessive heat inside the body (class 2), to lubricate dry symptoms (class 6), and to correct deficiencies (class 16).

FIRE

The human body needs fire to maintain normal body temperature, just like a room needs heat to be kept warm; hence, fire is essential to human health, which is why the Chinese call it "friendly fire." However, fire can also be a hostile energy when it originates from the five other atmospheric energies.

When heat bursts into flames, it becomes fire, and this can happen under two different circumstances. First, a person may be suffering from the common cold, with low fever at the beginning; but the fever may drag on and on, and finally the common cold develops into meningitis (inflammation of the membranes of the spinal cord or brain), because the heat that has built up in the body has burst into flames. Secondly, when a person is under stress for a prolonged period, he or she may accumulate internal heat that eventually bursts into flames to cause insomnia, lumbago, a cough, or asthma. When this happens, the Chinese call it "emotions transformed into fire," which will be discussed in more detail later.

When extreme summer heat turns into fire, the Chinese call it "summer heat transformed into fire." When cold turns into fire, they call it "cold transformed into fire." And when wind turns into fire, they call it "wind transformed into fire."

When the common cold develops into pneumonia, the Chinese say that it is due to "wind cold transformed into fire," because the common cold is

42

caused by "wind cold," and pneumonia is caused by fire. When a person displays twitching of the arms and legs as well as muscular spasms, with both eyes looking straight ahead, it is due to "wind transformed into fire." When a person displays fever, thirst, profuse perspiration, and a red face, it is due to "summer heat transformed into fire." When a person displays scorched lips, a dry tongue, and talking during sleep, it is due to "dampness transformed into fire." When a person starts coughing up blood, it's due to "dryness transformed into fire." And when one has a red tongue, sore throat, and sleeplessness, it's due to "cold transformed into fire."

It is the nature of fire to burn upwards and spread quickly, which is why when fire causes disease, the symptoms develop and worsen very rapidly. Such symptoms include high fever, severe headache, coma, vomiting of blood, and discharge of blood from the mouth. Since fire burns upwards, the symptoms caused by fire mostly occur in the upper part of the body. For instance, when stomach heat is transformed into fire, the symptoms include skin eruptions in the face, red and swollen eyes, and cankers on the tongue and in the mouth, all of which occur in the upper region.

Fire takes a heavy toll on both body fluids and body energy. Since fire burns upwards and in all directions, it opens up the pores all over the body, causing profuse perspiration. Fire can also cause bleeding, vomiting, and diarrhea, which take a heavy toll on body fluids. Similarly, fire is extreme heat that speeds up the rate of metabolism, so that the body will consume more energy than usual, which correspondingly reduces the quantity of energy left in the body. A typical example is a hyperfunctioning of the thyroid gland, known as hyperthyroidism, in which the basal-metabolic rate is increased, resulting in an increased demand for food to support this metabolic activity. Hyperthyroidism is caused by fire that consumes body fluids and eats up body energy. Although exceptions exist, most consumptive diseases are caused by fire, including hyperthyroidism, tuberculosis, fever, and many forms of cancer. Such diseases consume a great deal of body fluids and body energy that weaken the body.

Extreme heat turns into fire, and extreme fire produces toxic effects, which in Chinese medicine is called "toxic effects of fire" or "toxic fire" for short. How does fire produce toxic effects? At the beginning, fire consumes body fluids to create a shortage of fluids in the body. As time goes on, the shortage of body fluids may reach the stage where the body can no longer function normally, with the result that fire takes over and burns up each and every part of the body.

Symptoms caused by toxic fire are characterized by burning sensations with pain. Most cases of infections and inflammation fall within this category, including eye infections, kidney infections (nephritis), throat infections, inflammation of the lungs (pneumonia), boils, carbuncles, and urinary infections. All forms of cancer at the later stages, but lung cancer in particular, often display a cough, fever, chest pain, and vomiting of blood, which are due to the presence of toxic fire burning up body fluids.

43

Chemotherapy and radiation therapy used to treat cancer frequently produce toxic fire in the body, which is why many cancer patients complain about nausea and sore throat and other symptoms associated with toxic fire.

Although all five atmospheric energies can be transformed into fire to cause disease, this can happen more readily when body fluids are in short supply, which in Chinese medicine is called yin deficiency. When the five atmospheric energies are transformed into fire largely due to yin deficiency, it is called "fire of deficiency." This is in opposition to fire primarily caused by the strength of the five other atmospheric energies, which is called "fire of excess" in Chinese medicine. The symptoms normally caused by deficiency are night sweats, fear of the cold and wind, coughing up blood, forgetfulness, toothache, sore throat, dry mouth, dry throat, ringing in the ears, and sleeplessness. Some diseases in Western medicine caused by deficiency are iridocyclitis (inflammed iris and ciliary body), primary glaucoma, and trigeminal neuralgia.

How are herbs used to treat fire? In general, conditions that are due to "fire of excess" should be treated by the class of herbs to reduce excessive heat inside the body (class 2) and the class of herbs to induce bowel movements (class 8). In addition, each external hostile energy that has been transformed into fire should be treated accordingly. For instance, if wind has been transformed into fire, wind should be treated, and if dampness has been transformed into fire, dampness should be treated. Conditions due to "fire of deficiency" should be treated by the class of herbs to reduce excessive heat inside the body (class 2) and the class of herbs for lubricating dry symptoms (class 6).

EMOTIONS

In Chinese medicine, there are seven emotions: joy, anger, worry, thought, sadness, fear, and shock. The seven emotions do not cause disease under normal circumstances; they cause disease only when they are experienced suddenly and intensively or for a prolonged period of time. An excessive or extreme emotional state can cause a disorder of either energy or fire in a specific organ.

We often hear people say, "I was worried to death." Worry *can* cause disease, if not death. For instance, when we are worried about something, we are likely to lose our appetite or suffer indigestion.

In a study conducted in China, patients of neurasthenia (an illness characterized by chronic fatigue and sleeplessness) were divided into two groups, according to the state of their emotions. The patients who were considered emotionally fit were placed in the first group, while those who were considered unstable were placed in the second. Ninety-seven percent of the patients in the first group recovered from their illness, whereas only 5 percent in the second group recovered, during the same time period.

44

The Chinese believe that the emotions are connected to the internal organs. In Western medicine and psychology alike, a dichotomy exists between body and mind, but the same dichotomy does not exist in Chinese medicine. From the point of view of Chinese medicine, each internal organ is responsible for a specific emotion, and conversely, each emotion acts on a specific internal organ. Thus, the heart gives rise to joy, the liver gives rise to anger, the lungs give rise to worry and sadness, the spleen gives rise to thought, and the kidneys give rise to fear and shock. In other words, joy mirrors the state of the heart, anger mirrors the state of the liver, worry and sadness mirror the state of the lungs, and so on. Conversely, joy affects the state of the heart, anger affects the state of the liver, worry and sadness affect the state of the lungs, thought affects the state of the spleen, and fear and shock affect the state of the kidneys.

Excessive joy is harmful to the heart, because when a person is overjoyful, the energy of the heart will become too relaxed to concentrate, with the result that the person may suffer sleeplessness and forgetfulness. When extreme joy is transformed into "heart fire," the symptoms are abnormal laughter, ulcer on the tongue, and insanity.

Excessive anger is harmful to the liver, because when a person is very angry, the energy of the liver will rush upwards, causing the person to suffer from heavy sensations in the head and light sensations in the feet, ringing in the ears and deafness, headache, and pain in the ribs. When extreme anger is transformed into "liver fire," the common disorders are vomiting of blood, hypertension, acute conjunctivitis, epilepsy, and hyperthyroidism.

Excessive worry and sadness are harmful to the lungs, because when a person worries too much and feels sad for a prolonged period of time, the energy of the lungs becomes blocked up. As a result, the person may suffer from chronic inflammation of the nasal mucosa (chronic rhinitis), bronchial asthma, and inflammation of the stomach (gastritis). When extreme worry and sadness are transformed into "lungs fire," the symptoms are pain in the throat with red swelling, a dry nose, vomiting of blood, facial acne, asthma, a cough, and nosebleed.

Excessive thought is harmful to the spleen. When a person thinks too much, the energy of the spleen becomes congested, with the result that the person may suffer from chronic indigestion and diarrhea and suppression of menstruation in women. When extreme thought is transformed into "spleen fire," the symptoms are red and swollen lips, recurrent canker sores, bad breath, abdominal swelling, and frequent thirst.

Excessive fear and shock are harmful to the kidneys. When a person is in fear and shock, the energy of the kidneys becomes disordered, causing the person to suffer from night sweats, urination disorders, and impotence. When extreme fear and shock are transformed into "kidneys fire," the symptoms are bleeding gums, bone weakness, discharge of red urine, and diabetes.

45

How do we treat disorders caused by emotions? Basically by herbal tonics. When excessive joy causes harm to the heart, heart tonics should be used to treat the heart; when excessive anger causes harm to the liver, liver tonics should be used to treat the liver; when excessive worry and sadness cause harm to the lungs, lung tonics should be used to treat the lungs; when excessive thought causes harm to the spleen, spleen-pancreas tonics should be used to treat the spleen; when excessive fear and shock cause harm to the kidneys, kidney yang tonics and yin tonics should be used to treat the kidneys.

When extreme emotions cause fire in the internal organs, it should be treated by the class of herbs to reduce excessive heat inside the body (class 2), to lubricate dry symptoms (class 6), to reduce anxiety (class 14), and to correct deficiencies (class 16).

FATIGUE

When a person goes to see a doctor, he or she may be advised by the doctor to take it easy and rest for a few days, if the doctor believes that the illness is due to fatigue. However, Western doctors in general are not very clear about exactly how fatigue causes or intensifies disease. Chinese physicians, on the other hand, are more specific about the relationship between fatigue and disease.

According to Chinese medicine, five types of fatigue are harmful to health: Using the eyes for too long is harmful to the blood; lying for too long is harmful to energy; sitting for too long is harmful to muscles; standing for too long is harmful to bones; and walking for too long is harmful to tendons.

Excessive fatigue is particularly harmful to the spleen, as it can cause a disease known as "spleen deficiency." The symptoms are slightly cold hands and feet, abdominal swelling, being either underweight or overweight with a poor appetite, chronic diarrhea, indigestion, wanting to lie down, morning sickness during pregnancy, excessive menstrual bleeding, irregular menstruation, anemia, and a pale complexion.

Excessive sex also results in fatigue, and is particularly harmful to the kidneys, causing a disease known as "kidneys deficiency." The symptoms are hair loss, frequent miscarriage and menstrual pain in women, lumbago, toothache, ringing in the ears, diabetes, palpitations, fear of the cold, dizziness, shortness of breath, cold feet, frequent urination, impotence in men and infertility in women, and cold sensations in the genitals.

How do we use herbs in the treatment of fatigue? Fatigue due to excess labor is called "fatigue of excess" and should be treated by reducing the length and intensity of labor. On the other hand, fatigue due to internal deficiency occurs when someone always feels fatigued even though he or she may not be working hard at all. This type of fatigue is called "fatigue of deficiency." Since the spleen and kidneys are the two internal organs

46

most susceptible to the attack of fatigue, they both should be treated accordingly. When the spleen is affected by "fatigue of deficiency," blood, energy, spleen-pancreas, and stomach tonics should be used. When "fatigue of deficiency" affects the kidneys, energy tonics, kidney yang tonics, kidney yin tonics, liver tonics, and yin tonics should be used.

FOODS

How do foods cause disease? People in the West are familiar with the connection between sweet foods and diabetes, salt and hypertension, and saturated fats and heart disease. In Chinese medicine, however, food can cause disease in three different ways.

First, irregular eating habits may cause disorders to the digestive system. So, the general rule is that one should eat only when hungry, drink only when thirsty, and stop eating when 80 percent full. This is common sense, which requires no further explanation.

Second, eating the wrong foods under the wrong circumstances may cause or intensify certain disorders. For instance, if a person eats hot spicy foods, such as cayenne pepper, cloves, and garlic, while having a high fever, throat pain, constipation, or skin eruptions with red lesions, he or she is eating the wrong foods under the wrong circumstances, because such foods will intensify these symptoms. And when a person is ill, one menu may be beneficial whereas another menu may be harmful.

Third, eating foods that are inconsistent with one's physical type may also cause disease, because a specific food may be good for one physical type but bad for another. This means that the value of different foods should be judged according to each individual's physical type. If, for example, you frequently look pale and feel dizzy and fatigued, you undoubtedly have a low energy level; thus, you should avoid foods that may expend your energy more rapidly, such as carrots, dill seeds, garlic, and mustard seed.

3
How To Decoct and Take Herbs

METHODS OF DECOCTION

Traditionally, the Chinese have prepared herbs for consumption by decoction in the following manner to yield the best therapeutic effects.

First of all, the pot to be used for decoction should be made of something other than iron or bronze, in order to prevent chemical changes; usually, an earthenware pot is used instead. Place the herbs in the pot, add cold water just enough to cover all the herbs, and then add one more cup so that the water will be about a half an inch higher than the herbs. Stir a little bit and let the herbs soak in the water for about 20 minutes. Then start boiling the water; as soon as the water begins to boil, reduce the heat to low, both to keep the water from overflowing and to prevent its premature exhaustion. During the course of decoction, the pot should be covered and not opened too frequently in order to retain the volatile constituents of certain herbs.

If two or more herbs are to be decocted together as in a formula, the heavy or hard herbs, such as those consisting of wood or roots, should generally be decocted over low heat for 10 to 20 minutes first. This way, their constituents can become fully soluble in the boiling water; also, clinical experiences have shown that repeated decoction of heavy herbs for many types of usages produces good results. After the heavy and hard herbs have been boiled for 10 to 20 minutes, add the aromatic herbs, and then the very light herbs, which should be decocted for only about 5 minutes in order to prevent the evaporation of certain constituents.

It's important to note that decocting some toxic herbs for many hours over low heat may reduce their toxicity or completely eliminate it. Fortunately, as a rule, toxic herbs are processed by Chinese merchants before they are sold to herb shops.

The total decoction time depends upon the herbs being decocted. For example, herbs for inducing perspiration can be decocted over high heat for less than 10 minutes after the water starts boiling, whereas herbs for

49

strengthening the body, traditionally called tonics, can be decocted over low heat for as long as an hour.

When a Chinese patient gets a prescription from an herbalist, he or she usually brings it to an herb shop for filling. The clerk at the herb shop will place the herbs in small paper bags, with instructions for the contents of each bag to be decocted two to three times for oral administration. Normally, each decoction is to be taken all at once as one dosage, usually in 1 or 2 cups, and two dosages are taken a day.

METHODS OF TAKING HERBS

There is no best time for taking herbs, as it depends on which particular herbs you are taking and for which specific disorders. As a general rule, herbs that may disturb the digestive system and herbs for eye diseases should be taken after meals. Herbs for malaria should be taken 2 hours prior to onset. Herbs to induce sleep, as for insomnia, should be taken before bedtime. Herbs for acute symptoms can be taken anytime, whereas herbs for chronic diseases should be taken according to a fixed schedule on a regular basis. Herbs consumed as tonics to strengthen the body should be taken before meals. In addition, certain herbs can be drunk like tea many times a day without any fixed schedule.

The Chinese have this saying: "Withered plants will blossom and migratory birds will return every year on schedule." When they apply this principle to taking herbs, it means that those herbs should be taken regularly, according to a fixed schedule, usually every day at the same time.

When herbs are used to treat a disease in or above the chest, they should be taken after meals; however, when they are used to treat a disease below the heart, they should be taken before meals. When herbs are used to treat a disease of the arms and legs and the blood vessels, they should be taken on an empty stomach; but when they are used to treat a disease of the bones and marrow, they should be taken at night and after meals.

Certain herbs should be taken very warm while others taken cold, depending on the disease under treatment. Herbs taken to induce perspiration, as for the common cold, should be taken very warm or relatively hot. After taking such herbs, the patient should keep warm and perhaps have a little soup to reinforce the effects of the herbs. When herbs are taken to treat a hot disease, they should be taken cold; when herbs are taken to treat a cold disease, they should be taken hot. However, certain herbs can cause vomiting if taken hot, so these herbs should always be taken cold.

Some patients have a habit of taking herbs with tea for the sake of convenience, but this is definitely not advisable, and warm water should be drunk instead. For one thing, tea is obstructive, so it can obstruct the movements of herbs, thus reducing their effects. In the second place, tea has a cold energy that can interfere with the warm energy of the herbs being taken. And thirdly, tea contains caffeine and theophylline that can excite the central nervous system. When herbs for treating insomnia, for example, are taken with tea, these ingredients can cancel out the calming effects of the herbs.

DOSAGES OF HERBS

The quantity of herbs to be taken each time depends upon the effects of the specific herbs, the severity of the disease under treatment, the type of herbal formula, and the physical conditions of the patient. First of all, it's important to remember that some herbs are toxic while others are not, and that toxic herbs should be taken in smaller dosages than nontoxic herbs, and gradually increased to avoid drastic effects. Lighter herbs, such as those consisting of flowers and leaves, and aromatic herbs should generally be taken in smaller dosages, whereas heavy herbs can be taken in larger dosages. The dosages are always determined by the weight, as opposed to the volume, of the herbs.

It's best to treat a light or chronic disease with smaller dosages, and a severe or acute disease with larger dosages. This is because, according to Chinese medicine, body energy and disease are two opposing sides; they are each other's enemies, so to speak. And in a light disease, the disease is rather weak while body energy is still fairly strong, so that the body needs only a little help from the herbs to successfully resist the attack of the disease. In other words, in a light disease, life is not in danger and so one can take it easy in winning the battle over the disease; but in a severe disease, life may be in danger and the body needs more assistance from the herbs to resist the attack of the disease, which is why larger dosages of herbs are required.

Also, it's important to note that some herbs produce opposite effects when they are used in smaller or larger dosages. For example, when goldthread is used in smaller dosages, it can strengthen the stomach; but when it is used in larger dosages, it can dry and cause harm to the stomach.

Finally, the physical conditions of the patient, including body size, age, sex, and body strength, should be taken into account in determining dosages. Children and older patients should take smaller dosages than strong and middle-aged patients; stronger patients should take larger dosages than weaker patients; men should take larger dosages than women; and pregnant women and women right after childbirth should take smaller dosages than other women. In addition, generally larger dosages should be taken in the cold winter and smaller dosages should be taken in the hot summer.

4
The Herbs and Their Legends

For each of the herbs discussed in this chapter, information in the following categories is included.

Chinese: This is the Romanization of the name of the herb under discussion. Commonly called *pinyin*, it is also the Chinese pronunciation of the name of the herb.

Re: This is the reference number of the herb, based upon *An Encyclopedic Dictionary of Chinese Herbs*, compiled by the Jiangsu College of Traditional Chinese Medicine, and published in two volumes by the Shanghai Scientific Technology Press in 1977. This publication lists over 5,000 Chinese herbs, with their assigned reference numbers.

Common name: A Chinese herb may have more than one common name. However, the common names listed in this book are the ones most frequently used. The common name of an herb should not be used for identification purposes.

Family: In biology, this is used to refer to a major subdivision in the classification of plants and animals.

Chinese name: Chinese is an ideogramic language, which means that Chinese words represent ideas or objects, rather than speech sounds, as in English. So, when Chinese words are used to name an herb, the words represent an idea or ideas; the Chinese name of an herb listed here is usually the English translation of those ideas.

Scientific name: This is the scientific or botanical name of the herb under discussion.

Pharmaceutical name: This is the pharmaceutical name of the herb. It normally consists of two or more words—with the first word representing the part of the plant being used as the herb, and the remaining word or words denoting the overall plant. For example, "radix ginseng" means that the root of the plant is used as the herb, because "radix" means root; "ginseng" refers to the plant called Panax Ginseng C. A. Mey.

53

Part used: Different parts of a plant can be used as herbs with different functions, such as leaves, roots, stems, fruit, or seeds.

Dosage: The indicated dosages are for one-day consumption for an adult, when the herb is decocted and used as a single ingredient. Dosages should be reduced by half for children between 6 and 13 years old, by one third for children between 3 and 5 years old, and by one quarter for children under 3 years old.

Flavor: An herb may taste sweet, bitter, pungent, salty, sour, light, or constrictive.

Energy: An herb may be cold, cool, warm, hot, or neutral in energy.

Class: There is a total of 20 classes of herbs; a given herb can belong to one or more classes. (The classes are described in pages 19–30.)

Meridians: There is a total of 12 meridians through which herbs may travel after they have been digested. When an herb travels through a meridian, it means the herb is acting on that meridian and related organ.

Actions: The actions of herbs are important to remember, because they often give us evidence for their applications.

Indications: These are the symptoms and diseases that are treated by a given herb. However, a disorder may be due to different causes, which means that it should be treated differently; for this reason, the actions of herbs should be taken into account before the herbs are used to treat the disorders in this category.

Notes: This includes additional information about the herb in question, including modern experiments.

ELEVEN LONGEVITY HERBS

Medicinal Cornel Fruit (Sour Mountain Date, *Shanzhuyu*) and Morinda Root (Never-Withering-and-Falling, *Bajitian*)

Throughout Chinese history, most Chinese emperors lived a relatively short life, partly because of their involvements in hectic politics and partly because of their excessive indulgence in sex. Both took their toll, physically and emotionally, at least from the point of view of Chinese medicine. However, an emperor named Qian Long of the Manchu Dynasty (1644–1911) was recorded to have lived the longest life of all the Chinese emperors prior to his time, dying at the age of 89. Emperor Qian Long was said to have frequently boasted about the secret methods he used to achieve longevity, and had called himself "the long-life emperor."

That Qian Long had managed to stay youthful and had lived a long life is a historical fact. The British ambassador to China at that time was said to have written something like this in his diary, "When I met Emperor Qian Long, he was already at the age of 83, but he looked as if he was only 60 years old. He was in perfect good health and surpassed young men in energy and spirits." Many Chinese physicians have attributed Qian Long's

54

longevity to his regular consumption of many herbs, but most notably, medicinal cornel fruit and morinda root.

The fruit of medicinal cornel looks like a date, tastes sour, and is found mostly in the mountains, which is why the Chinese call it "sour mountain date."

But what makes this sour mountain date capable of promoting longevity? The story behind this is that the flowers of this plant appear as early as May, but its fruit do not become ripe until November, which means that it takes a longer period of time than other plants to bear fruit. Moreover, in November when most other plants have died, the sour mountain date has not only survived, but its fruit are hanging from it elegantly. The fact that it takes a long time for the sour mountain date to bear fruit signifies that the fruit must have a certain element of long life in them, and the fact that this plant can resist the assault of severe winter cold means that there must be a quality of toughness in it.

The fruit of medicinal cornel was used as the "king ingredient" in a celebrated Chinese herbal formula, called "the eight-flavoured tablets," during the third century A.D. This formula was used to treat many serious disorders, including diabetes, chronic nephritis, and sexual weaknesses. A "king ingredient" means that the ingredient plays a very important role in the formula. A report prepared by the National Peking Research Institute indicates that the fruit of medicinal cornel can promote urination and lower blood pressure for many hours.

What follows are standard, modern descriptions of this herb.

Chinese: *Shanzhuyu* (Sour Mountain Date).
Re: 0370.
Common name: medicinal cornel fruit.
Family: Cornaceae.
Chinese name: wild date (so named because of its shape like a date).
Scientific name: Cornus officinalis Sieb et Zucc.
Pharmaceutical name: Fructus Corni.
Part used: fruit.
Dosage: 5 g.
Flavor: sour.
Energy: slightly warm.
Class: 17, herbs to constrict and obstruct movements.
Meridians: liver and kidneys.
Actions: to tone up the liver and kidneys, constrict semen, and check perspiration.

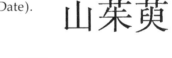

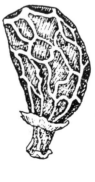

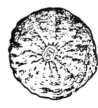

55

Indications: seminal emission, excessive perspiration, lumbago, dizziness, ringing in ears, and insomnia.

Notes: Experiments have shown *shanzhuyu* to be effective in inhibiting gastrointestinal peristalsis and in reducing blood sugar. Since this herb is obstructive, it is not recommended for those with constipation.

Shanzhuyu and *jinyingzi*, which will be discussed later, are both constrictive with the effects of tonification. So, they can be used to treat seminal emission, seminal sliding, enuresis, excessive urination, excessive menstrual flow, and vaginal discharge due to kidney deficiency.

Shanzhuyu can be decocted with *renshen* (radix ginseng), which will be discussed later, to treat patients with extremely cold sensations after profuse perspiration.

To treat insomnia, fry 20 g *shanzhuyu* quickly over low heat until it is dry, grind into powder to soak in 5 cups of wine, and seal in bottle. Leave for one month, shaking the bottle once a day. Then strain it to drink the wine, twice a day, in the morning and in the evening. To treat other diseases, decoct 10 g *shanzhuyu* in water for consumption in a standard manner (see Chapter 3).

*   *   *

Morinda root is called "never-withering-and-falling" in Chinese, because it is a creeping vine that hangs on persistently, and "never withering and falling" means longevity in Chinese. The root of this plant, which is used for medicinal purposes, contains vitamin C and carbohydrates.

Chinese: *Bajitian* (Never-Withering-and-Falling). 巴戟天
Re: 1034.
Common name: morinda root.
Family: Rubiaceae.
Chinese name: morinda root.
Scientific name: Morinda officinalis How.

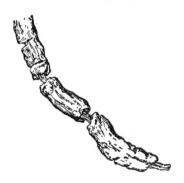

Pharmaceutical name: Radix Morindae Officinalis.
Part used: root.
Dosage: 7 to 18 g.
Flavor: pungent and sweet.
Energy: warm.
Class: 16, herbs to correct deficiencies.
Meridians: kidneys.

Actions: to warm up the kidneys, strengthen yang, and strengthen tendons and bones.

Indications: kidney yang deficiency, impotence, lumbago, dizziness, and ringing in ears.

Notes: *Bajitian* is effective for treating impotence, lumbago, and cold-damp rheumatism due to kidney yang deficiency.

56

Glutinous Rehmannia (New Place, Old Place)

A Chinese government official in the Ming Dynasty (1368–1644), known as Mayor Lin, was said to have fathered a baby girl at the age of 104, and he was believed to be in the habit of taking glutinous rehmannia. The Chinese have a famous riddle: "I have visited a new place and returned to an old one simultaneously, what herb am I?" The answer is: "I am glutinous rehmannia." When glutinous rehmannia is used in raw form, it is called "new place," because the Chinese ideograms for raw glutinous rehmannia and "new place" are identical; but when rehmannia is processed by steaming and drying in the sun, it is called "old place," because the Chinese ideograms for processed glutinous rehmannia and "old place" are identical. The Chinese traditionally process raw glutinous rehmannia by steaming it 10 times and drying it in the sun nine times, in order to make it shiny and black as if it were painted with black ink. But why do the Chinese bother to go to such great lengths in processing it? There is a good reason underlying their efforts.

Raw glutinous rehmannia can reduce heat in the blood, whereas processed glutinous rehmannia can treat blood deficiency. Thus, in Chinese herbalism, the raw and the processed forms of glutinous rehmannia are regarded as two entirely different herbs. They belong to two different classes and there's a world of difference between them in terms of their clinical uses.

A report published in the *Chinese Medical Journal* indicates that raw glutinous rehmannia has been shown to be effective in the treatment of rheumatic and rheumatoid arthritis. Also, glutinous rehmannia and licorice have been shown to be a good combination. A report published in the *Medical Technology Reporter* indicates that in the treatment of bronchial asthma, injections of processed glutinous rehmannia and processed licorice have produced very positive results. Another report, published in the *New Pharmacological Journal*, indicates obvious improvements in cases of contagious hepatitis treated by injections of raw glutinous rehmannia and raw licorice.

Chinese: *Shengdi* (New Place). 生地
Re: 5370.
Common name: glutinous rehmannia (raw).
Family: Berberidaceae.
Chinese name: fresh earth's yellowness (literal translation).
Scientific name: Rehmannia glutinosa Libosch.
Pharmaceutical name: Radix Rehmanniae.

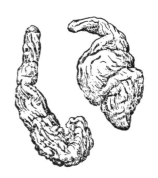

57

Part used: dried tuberous root.

Dosage: 10 to 90 g.

Flavor: sweet and bitter.

Energy: cold.

Classes: herbs to reduce excessive heat inside the body (class 2) and herbs for lubricating dry symptoms (class 6).

Meridians: heart, liver, and kidneys.

Actions: to increase yin energy to a moderate degree, bring down fire, cool down the blood, lubricate the intestine, and produce fluids.

Indications: sore throat, vomiting of blood, coughing up blood, nosebleed, discharge of urine containing blood, and diabetes.

Notes: Experiments have shown *shengdi* to be an effective heart tonic and an effective coagulant.

Shengdi is sticky and contains moisture. So, when it is decocted with other herbs, it should be decocted first for 10 minutes before adding the other herbs.

Chinese: *Shudihuang* (Old Place).

Re: 5517.

Common name: steamed glutinous rehmannia.

Family: Scrophulariaceae.

Chinese name: cooked earth's yellowness (literal translation).

Scientific name: Rehmannia glutinosa Libosch.

Pharmaceutical name: Radix Rehmanniae praeparatae.

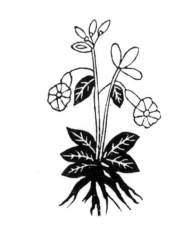

Part used: tuberous root.

Dosage: 20 g.

Flavor: sweet.

Energy: slightly warm.

Class: 16, herbs to correct deficiencies.

Meridians: liver and kidneys.

Actions: to tone up blood, water kidneys, nourish yin, and make grey hair return to former color.

Indications: blood deficiency, grey hair, ringing in ears, night sweats, vaginal bleeding, diabetes, and seminal emission.

Notes: Experiments have shown that *shudihuang* can protect the liver and reduce blood sugar.

Shudihuang is good for kidney yin deficiency with dizziness and vertigo. It is an effective blood tonic and is also effective for the arrestment of bleeding due to blood deficiency, and can thus be used to treat such symptoms as palpitations, excessive menstrual flow, and blood in urine.

58

Matrimony Vine (Thorny Stalk Seed, *Gouqizi*)

There is a story about a Chinese traveller who, while passing through a village called Xihe, happened to witness a young lady beating an old man with grey hair all over his head. The young lady looked about 15 or 16 years old, and the old man somewhere between 80 and 90. The traveller asked the young lady why she was beating the old man, and she explained that she was his granddaughter and she was angry with him for failing to take his longevity herbs. That was why he looked so old, she said. The traveller asked her age and was told that she was 372 years old. Rather taken aback, he asked her how she had managed to live that long, and she replied that she consumed matrimony vine all year around.

China's greatest herbalist, Shih-Chen Li, who wrote the celebrated *Outline of Materia Medica,* published in 1578, pointed out in this book that the people in the village of Nan-Qiu were in the habit of eating matrimony vine and that a very high percentage of them lived a long life. And a famous Chinese poet in the Tang Dynasty (618–907) by the name of Yu-Xi Liu wrote a poem in praise of the wonderful effects of matrimony vine, which said that even the water from a well near the plant can make people live a long life.

In fact, matrimony vine is not only good for longevity, but it is often associated with beauty as well. For instance, a Chinese writer reported that he knew a beautiful woman from a wealthy family who had always made it a point to drink matrimony vine tea and eat the seeds every day, which was why, he said, she looked 20 years younger than her age.

Matrimony vine is a trailing shrub with thorny stalks. Its seeds are the most valuable part for medicinal purposes, although the roots of this plant are beneficial as well.

Another story relates how a scholar spotted some beautiful flowers on the plant, so out of curiosity he began to dig out the roots. To his amazement, the roots were shaped like two dogs bound together. But he washed them anyway and boiled them in water. After having eaten the roots for a few days, the scholar all of a sudden felt very light in his body, as if he could fly away.

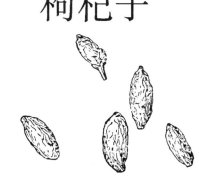

Chinese: *Gouqizi* (Thorny Stalk Seed).

Re: 3163.

Common name: matrimony vine fruit.

Family: Solanaceae.

Chinese name: aspen-willow fruit (so named because this herb is as thorny as an aspen, its stems resemble those of a willow, and its fruit is used).

Scientific name: Lycium barbarum L.

59

Pharmaceutical name: Fructus Lycii.
Part used: ripe fruit.
Dosage: 6 g.
Flavor: sweet.
Energy: neutral.
Class: 16, herbs to correct deficiencies.
Meridians: liver, lungs, and kidneys.
Actions: to tone up kidneys, nourish the liver, nourish blood, and sharpen vision.
Indications: blood deficiency with dizziness and blurred vision, lumbago, seminal emission, and diabetes.
Notes: Experiments have shown that *gouqizi* can protect the liver and reduce blood sugar.

Gouqizi can tonify the kidneys. It is good for dizziness, vertigo, and lumbago, due to kidney deficiency, as well as for dizziness and vertigo, due to liver deficiency. It is also good for nourishing the liver to sharpen vision.

Gouqizi can be decocted with *juhua* to nourish the liver and sharpen vision. This combination is considered very beneficial for people suffering from dizziness and blurred vision.

Momordica Fruit (Arhat Fruit, *Luohanguo*)

Momordica fruit is one of the few fruits that cannot be eaten until it is dried by fire. For the last few centuries, this fruit has almost exclusively been a product of the province of Guangxi in southern China. The people of this region have called this fruit "longevity fruit" because they have believed that a prolonged consumption of it would make people live a long life. This fruit is said to resemble the stomach of a Buddha, which is why its official Chinese name is "arhat fruit," since "arhat" refers to a Buddhist who has attained Nirvana.

Momordica fruit has traditionally been used for a number of common ailments, such as cough with sputum, constipation, chronic laryngitis, hoarseness, and chronic bronchitis. But it has also recently emerged as an important herb in the curing and prevention of cancer. According to a Japanese report, this fruit contains an unnamed substance that makes it taste 300 times sweeter than ordinary sugar. Although it tastes so sweet, the Chinese nevertheless believe that it is good for diabetes.

Chinese: *Luohanguo* (Arhat Fruit).　　　　羅漢果
Re: 2806.
Common name: fruit of Grosvenor Momordica.
Family: Cucurbitaceae.
Chinese name: big fellow's fruit.

60

Scientific name: Momordica grosvenori Swingle.

Pharmaceutical name: Fructus Momordicae.

Part used: fruit.

Dosage: 10 to 16 g.

Flavor: sweet.

Energy: cool.

Classes: herbs to suppress coughing and reduce sputum (class 10) and herbs to induce bowel movements (class 8).

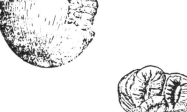

Meridians: lungs and spleen.

Actions: to clear lungs and lubricate intestines.

Indications: whooping cough, cough with sputum fire, and constipation due to dry blood.

Oriental Arborvitae Seed (*Baiziren*)

A notorious Chinese emperor in the Qin Dynasty (221–207 B.C.) called himself "the first emperor of China," meaning that, after his death, his son would be the second emperor and his grandson the third, and on and on without interruption. Not only had the emperor built the Great Wall to head off possible foreign invasion from the North, but he had also kept over 3,000 concubines in his palace to satisfy his fantasies. But no sooner had the emperor died than his palace was burned down and the empire he had built came to a total collapse. All the concubines either escaped or were sent away from the palace by the new conqueror, and one was later found in the woods.

After this concubine escaped from the palace, she hid in the woods, where there was little to eat. After a while, she met an old man, who advised her to eat Oriental arborvitae seeds. Since they were not pleasing to the taste, she hesitated at first, but finally came to realize that she had no choice. And so, she began to eat them, gradually becoming used to their taste. As it turned out, she developed great strength in resisting the severe winter cold as well as the extreme summer heat.

It wasn't until a century and a half later that a group of hunters found her in the woods; she was naked and had long black hair, and was seen escaping as fast as a monkey. The hunters were very curious and ran after her in pursuit. Once they finally captured her, they questioned her and were shocked to find that the black-haired woman used to be a concubine of the first emperor of China, and that she was now 200 years old.

From the point of view of modern medicine, Oriental arborvitae seed contains 14 percent fat, volatile oil, and saponin. It can reduce cholesterol level and prevent cardiovascular diseases.

61

Chinese: _Baiziren_ (Oriental Arborvitae Seed).
Re: 3154.
Common name: Oriental arborvitae kernel.
Family: Cupressaceae
Chinese name: lateral cypress kernel (so named because its leaves are flat and grow laterally).
Scientific name: Biota orientalis (L.) Endl.
Pharmaceutical name: Semen Biotae.
Part used: ripe kernel.
Dosage: 6 g.
Flavor: sweet.
Energy: neutral.
Class: 14, herbs to reduce anxiety.
Meridians: heart and spleen.

柏子仁

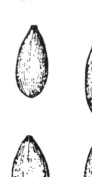

Actions: to secure the heart, check perspiration, lubricate dryness, and induce bowel movements.

Indications: insomnia, palpitations, constipation, and night sweats.

Notes: Experiments have shown that _baiziren_ can sedate and inhibit.

Sesame (Barbarian's Hemp, _Heizhima_)

A Chinese woman in ancient China was said to have consumed sesame for more than 80 years on end, which made her live to over 90 years of age, and still look like a young lady. At 90, she could still walk 300 miles a day, and run as fast as a deer.

A Chinese document relates that sesame can be boiled and made into tablets as big as bullets. By taking one tablet each day for one year, you will get a shiny complexion. By taking the same dosage for 2 years, the grey hair will go away; for 3 years, lost teeth will grow back; for 4 years, you will have complete freedom from disease; for 5 years, you will be able to run as fast as a horse; and for life, you will achieve longevity. From the point of view of modern medicine, sesame contributes to longevity primarily because it contains vitamin E.

Sesame can also increase the beauty of the skin, and the Chinese often make use of a combination of sesame and rice powder as a beauty formula. First, fry sesame in an oil-free pan, and, after a while, add a little water and mix thoroughly. Next, strain the sesame, and add a little rice powder to the sesame fluid. Then bring the fluid to a boil over low heat. Remove from heat and add a little honey or sugar or other condiments to taste.

The Chinese believe that the skin can be made beautiful, not by vegetables or fruits alone, but also by an adequate amount of vegetable oils, particularly sesame. The combination of sesame and rice powder is also

62

effective for treating constipation, which is a symptom that needs to be corrected if the skin is to become beautiful.

Sesame is called barbarian's hemp in Chinese, because it looks like hemp and it was originally imported from a foreign country on the western border of China by a Chinese general named Zhang Qian, when he was sent by the Chinese emperor to conquer that country in 119 B.C. It must be pointed out that the Chinese regarded all foreigners as barbarians during that period of Chinese history.

Chinese: *Heizhima* (Barbarian's Hemp).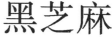
Re: 4955.
Common name: sesame.
Family: Pedaliaceae.
Chinese name: wild sesame.
Scientific name: Sesamum indicum L.
Pharmaceutical name: Semen Sesami.
Part used: seed.
Dosage: 3 to 12 g.
Flavor: sweet.
Energy: neutral.
Classes: herbs for lubricating dry symptoms (class 6) and herbs to correct deficiencies (class 16).
Meridians: liver and kidneys.

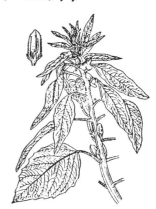

Actions: to tone up the liver and kidneys, and lubricate the five viscera.
Indications: liver-kidney deficiency, headaches, dizziness, ringing in the ears, constipation, and shortage of milk secretion in women.

Notes: *Heizhima* can tonify and nourish the liver and the kidneys. It is an effective herb for blurred vision and dizziness, ringing in the ears, and numbness of the arms and legs. It is associated with yin deficiency of the liver and the kidneys.

Slender Acanthopanax Root Bark
(Thorny Ginseng, *Wujiapi*)

According to a story told by China's most celebrated herbalist, Shih-Chen Li, half a dozen Chinese politicians and scholars prior to his time had lived to be over 300 years old as a result of consuming slender acanthopanax root bark soaked in rice wine, traditionally known as "thorny ginseng wine." Legends of this sort are taken so seriously by some Chinese people that one famous poet declared that he would "rather have a taste of thorny ginseng wine than be in possession of a cartful of gold."

When I visited China in 1983, I bought a few bottles of liquid made from this plant, and the label said, "good for neurasthenia, insomnia, many dreams, forgetfulness, dizziness, poor appetite, palpitation, coronary heart

63

disease, angina pectoris, and a prolonged consumption will cure leukopenia caused by physiotherapy and chemotherapy, and will slow down aging."

A report prepared by the Seventh Shanghai Pharmaceutical Factory said that of the 43 cases of leukopenia treated with this herb, 70.4 percent showed effective results, with a rise in white blood cells to normal within an average of 2 weeks. Among the patients treated, 37 cases were caused by chemotherapy and radiation of tumors, three cases were caused by hypersplenism, and three cases were due to other causes. The treatment involved an oral administration of 3.6 g of this herb each day, for a period of 3 to 15 days. It was also indicated that the treatment showed better results in those cases caused by chemotherapy, and among them, two cases underwent a marrow test, which showed signs of proliferation. And according to a statistical report compiled by 10 Chinese hospitals, of the 113 cases of tumor patients with leukopenia caused by chemotherapy and radiation treated by this herb, 13.7 percent showed obviously effective results, with an overall effective rate of 74.5 percent. In another report, 100 cases of chronic tracheitis were treated with this herb. The results showed improvements in symptoms, in physical strength, and in frequency of attack, with the effect of increasing the function of the adrenal cortex.

Slender acanthopanax root bark comes from a shrub with many fine thorns on small branches, and belongs to the same family as Chinese ginseng, which is why the Chinese call it "thorny ginseng."

Chinese: *Wujiapi* (Thorny Ginseng).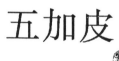
Re: 0767.
Common name: Acanthopanax root bark.
Family: Araliaceae.
Chinese name: five plus bark.
Scientific name: Acanthopanax gracilistylus W. W. Smith.
Pharmaceutical name: Cortex Acanthopanacis Radicis.
Part used: dry root bark.
Dosage: 6 to 12 g.
Flavor: pungent.
Energy: warm.
Class: 3, herbs to counteract rheumatism.
Meridians: liver and kidneys.

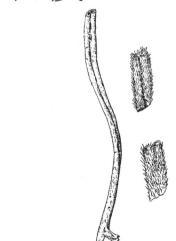

Actions: to remove wind and dampness, and strengthen bones and tendons.
Indications: rheumatism, beriberi, and weak limbs.

64

Notes: Experiments have shown *wujiapi* to be an effective heart tonic, as it can produce adrenocortical hormones, and also to be an effective herb for the relief of pain and rheumatism.

Wujiapi is especially effective in treating rheumatism in the lower half of the body due to dampness.

Sweet Apricot (*Tianxingren*) and Water Lily (Chicken Head Kernel, *Qianshi*)

A 60-year-old woman in the Wen Feng Commune suffered from a severe illness and was very overweight. Seeing that nothing could help her, her family started preparing her funeral. Meanwhile, an old Chinese doctor of traditional Chinese medicine told her to grind 450 g of sweet apricot and 450 g of water lily into a fine powder and to take the powder regularly. No sooner had she finished all the powder, than the woman recovered from her illness; continuing to take this powder, she was free from illness thereafter. The water lily fruit looks like the head of a chicken, which is why the Chinese call it "chicken head kernel."

There are two kinds of apricot kernel: bitter apricot kernel, called *kuxingren*, and sweet apricot kernel, called *tianxingren. Tianxingren* is larger than *kuxingren. Kuxingren* can expel sputum, suppress coughing, and lubricate the intestines, and is good for coughing and asthma and abundant sputum due to the common cold, as well as for constipation. *Tianxingren* can lubricate the lungs, suppress coughing, and make the intestines smooth; it is better for a chronic cough or a dry cough without sputum due to yin deficiency of the lungs.

In his celebrated classic, entitled *One Thousand Ounces Gold Classic,* published in 682, Sun Shu Mao (581–682) presented a formula for longevity called "sweet apricot mixture." You fry 5 kg of sweet apricot kernel quickly over low heat until dry, grind it into powder, and immerse it in rice wine. Next, you strain it and mix the liquid with 2.5 kg of honey to make a 7.5 kg mixture, which you boil over low heat again, until it becomes as thick as jelly. Then you put it in a container and seal it tightly. Take 20 to 35 g of this liquid per dosage to recover from an illness and achieve longevity.

Chinese: *Tianxingren* (Sweet Apricot). **Re:** 4495.

甜杏仁

Common name: sweet apricot seed.
Family: Rosaceae.
Chinese name: sweet apricot seed (so named because it tastes sweet).
Scientific name: Prunus armeniaca Linne.
Pharmaceutical name: Semen Armeniacae Dulcis.

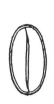
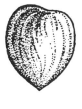

65

Part used: ripe seed.
Dosage: 10 g.
Flavor: sweet.
Energy: neutral.
Classes: herbs for lubricating dry symptoms (class 6) and herbs to suppress cough and reduce sputum (class 10).
Meridians: lungs and large intestine.
Actions: to lubricate lungs, expel sputum, suppress cough, and relieve asthma.
Indications: dry cough, asthma, and constipation.

Chinese: *Kuxingren* (Bitter Apricot).
Re: 2240.
Common name: bitter apricot kernel.
Family: Rosaceae.
Chinese name: bitter apricot kernel.
Scientific names: Prunus armeniaca L. var. ansu Maxim, prunus sibirica L, Prunus mandshurica (Maxim) Koehne, and Prunus armeniaca L.
Pharmaceutical name: Semen Armeniacae Amarum.
Part used: ripe kernel.
Dosage: 6 g.
Flavor: bitter.
Energy: warm.
Class: 10, herbs to suppress cough and reduce sputum.
Meridians: lungs and large intestine.

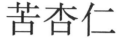

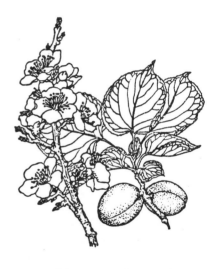

Actions: to suppress cough, expel sputum, expand lungs, and calm down asthma.
Indications: cough in the common cold, asthma with copious sputum, and constipation due to exhaustion of fluids.
Notes: Bitter apricot is slightly toxic. It contains cyanic glycosides that can suppress cough. Experiments have shown it to be effective for suppression of cough and also for asthma.

Chinese: *Qianshi* (Water Lily).
Re: 2183.
Common name: gorgon fruit.
Family: Nymphaceae.
Chinese name: gorgon fruit.
Scientific name: Euryale ferox Salisb.

66

Pharmaceutical name: Semen Euryales.
Part used: kernel.
Dosage: 6 to 10 g.
Flavor: sweet.
Energy: neutral.
Class: 17, herbs to constrict and obstruct movements.
Meridians: spleen and kidneys.
Actions: to strengthen the spleen, benefit the kidneys, solidify semen, and relieve diarrhea.
Indications: diarrhea due to spleen deficiency, seminal emission, and vaginal discharge.
Notes: *Qianshi* is obstructive and thus should be avoided by those with constipation.

Tuber of Multiflower Knotweed
(He's Black Hair, *Heshouwu*)

In 812, a 56-year-old man by the name of He was pruning his trees when two plants a few metres apart suddenly caught his attention. He thought it was very strange that the vines of these plants were crossing each other not unlike a man and a woman embracing each other in love. "There's got to be a good reason for these plants to be doing this kind of thing," he thought. He then dug out the roots of the plants and brought them home to cook and eat as food.

He had been so weak since childhood that he had never married. However, after consuming the roots for seven days, he began to have a desire for marriage. After consuming the roots for a few months, he began to feel much stronger; and after one year of consumption, his grey hair had all returned to black, and he began to look like a young man. At that point, He got married and then fathered a baby boy. Both the father and the son lived to over 130 years of age. The Chinese have called tuber of multiflower knotweed "He's black hair" ever since.

From the point of view of modern medicine, the effects of tuber of multiflower knotweed are similar to those of an adrenocortical hormone. In a medical experiment, two groups of animals were placed in a $-5°$ C refrigerator for $17\frac{1}{2}$ hours; before being placed in the refrigerator, one group was fed the herb for two weeks. The results showed that 32.3 percent of the animals in the group fed the herb died compared with the 67.7 percent death rate in the other group. In another experiment on the treatment of chronic tracheitis, one group of patients was treated by a standard herbal formula while another group was treated by the same herbal formula plus tuber of multiflower knotweed. The second group showed obviously better results, with both local symptoms and fear of wind and cold, cold sensations in the back, and shortness of breath considerably improved.

Chinese: *Heshouwu* (Mr. He's Black Hair). Re: 2310.

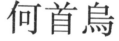

Common name: multiflower knot-weed tuber.

Family: Polygonaceae.

Chinese name: Mr. He's black hair.

Scientific name: Polygonum multiflorum Thunb.

Pharmaceutical name: Radix Polygoni Multiflori.

Part used: tuberous root.

Dosage: 10 to 25 g.

Flavor: bitter and sweet.

Energy: slightly warm.

Class: 16, herbs to correct deficiencies.

Meridians: liver and kidneys.

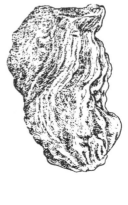

Actions: to tone up the liver and kidneys, and to benefit semen and blood.

Indications: seminal emission, vaginal discharge, lumbago, and premature grey hair.

Notes: According to experiments, *heshouwu* can treat fatty liver, increase red blood cells, and reduce blood fat.

AGRIMONY (RED-CROWNED CRANE'S HERB, *XIANHECAO*)

One summer two Chinese officials were making a long trip to Peking to take a national examination for promotion. Seeing that time was almost running out, they hastened their journey, only to find themselves in a desert without any village in sight. They were hungry and thirsty and physically exhausted, but they could find neither water to drink, food to eat, nor a place to rest. One of the officials suddenly developed a nosebleed, and the bleeding wouldn't stop, so his fellow traveller ripped a sheet of paper from an old book and squeezed it into his friend's nose. But it was in vain, as the blood continued to flow from his nose.

The official with the nosebleed said, "I wish I had some water." "Where could I possibly get water for you?" responded his nervous friend. "We are on a wide desert now. We're in dire straits. I wish someone would help us."

At that moment, a bird few past them with a loud cry. The official with the nosebleed looked up and saw a red-crowned crane circling over his head. "Dear bird, I wish I could borrow your wings to fly out of this desert," shouted the official, with both arms outstretched and his mouth wide open. Shocked by the official's loud shouting, the red-crowned crane suddenly opened its beak and a blade of grass dropped from it to the

68

ground. The official picked it up and murmured with a smile, "Even if I can't borrow your wings, I can still use this grass to moisten my mouth for some relief." And so, he put the grass in his mouth and started chewing it as if it were a piece of gum. Oddly enough, the nosebleed stopped after a short while, and both officials started jumping with joy. "The bird gave us a magic grass," one of them said jokingly.

The two Chinese officials made it to the examination hall in the capital just in time for the examination, and both of them passed and got promoted. When the two officials got together again some time later, they recalled the event on the desert and began to wonder about the grass that stopped the nosebleed. They started making inquiries about the name of the grass, but no herbalists knew anything about it. The two then drew pictures of the grass from their recollections and ordered their subordinates to search for it.

Finally, many years later, the grass was found growing along some hillsides. It was a perennial herb with long soft hairs over the entire plant. Discovering that the plant still had no name, the officials named it after the red-crowned crane.

Chinese: *Xianhecao* (Red-Crowned Crane's Herb). 仙鶴草

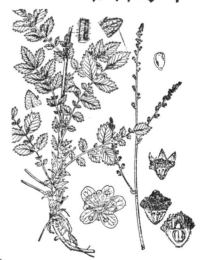

Re: 1372.

Common name: agrimony.

Family: Rosaceae.

Chinese name: red-crowned crane plant (literal translation).

Scientific name: Agrimonia pilosa Ledeb.

Pharmaceutical name: Herba Agrimoniae.

Part used: whole plant.

Dosage: 30 g.

Flavor: bitter.

Energy: neutral.

Class: 12, herbs to regulate blood.

Meridians: lung, spleen, stomach, and large intestine.

Actions: to constrict and arrest bleeding.

Indications: vomiting of blood, coughing up blood, nosebleeds, and vaginal bleeding.

Notes: Since *xianhecao* is obstructive, it should be avoided by those with constipation.

Experiments have shown that *xianhecao* can increase and protect blood platelets, and that it is an effective coagulant and can arrest bleeding (as a hemostatic).

69

Agrimony is an important Chinese herb used for the arrestment of bleeding, and its effects have been proven by modern research. In one study, 20 cases of bleeding, including bleeding from external causes, and bleeding caused by intracranial and thoracic and abdominal surgeries, were treated by the hemostatic powder made from this herb. The results of this study showed that the bleeding stopped within 1 to 2 minutes in all cases. Agrimony produced in the Soviet Union has been found to contain plenty of tannin and a small quantity of vitamin K-1, both of which are believed to be responsible for the hemostatic effects of the herb.

ANTIPYRETIC DICHROA (MOUNT ETERNITY, *CHANGSHAN*)

On a mountain in China called Mount Eternity, there was an old temple where a poor monk lived. This monk was so poor that he had to go all the way to a village to beg for food.

One day the monk was attacked by malaria, and he experienced intermittent fever and chills nearly once every day thereafter. He had lost a great deal of weight as a result of the malaria, and had come to a point where he could hardly walk. But the monk was so poor that he couldn't even consider seeking medical treatment.

One day the monk had gone to the village to beg for food as usual, but by noon had met with no success, and his stomach was rumbling like crazy. The monk thought to himself, "What will happen to me when the malaria strikes again this afternoon? How can I sustain the attack without eating anything?" With this thought in his head, the monk had come to knock at yet another door. But the poor fellow who answered said, "We do not have enough food to feed ourselves, so how can we feed you? We cooked some plant roots and started eating them, but then all of us started vomiting. If you are really hungry, you can try them." Feeling that he had no choice, the monk gobbled up all the plant roots on the table and left.

Oddly enough, the monk did not vomit nor did he experience any other discomfort. After walking a short distance, he sat down on some grass to take a sunbath while waiting for the onset of the malaria. He waited and waited for many hours, until by sunset, not only had the malaria not struck, but the monk felt unusually good and comfortable.

A few days passed, but the malaria still did not attack him. The monk was quite excited by the prospect of complete recovery. But, unfortunately, a month later, the malaria recurred.

Wondering if there was any correlation between eating the roots and his temporary recovery, the monk rushed back to the poor fellow's house who had given him the roots. He asked him what the roots were, and the fellow, still angry, responded, "Those were the roots my stupid son dug up on the mountain that made all of us sick for so many days." "Could you ask your son to lead me to the plants?" requested the monk.

70

And so, the poor fellow's son guided the monk to the mountain, where they found plenty of these plants growing on the ground. The plant turned out to be a deciduous shrub, with round stalks and branches, usually found growing on wet ground in the mountains. The monk dug out the roots and brought them home to cook and eat. The next day, after eating the roots, the malaria did not attack him. After continuing to eat them for a few more days, the monk found that he was totally free of the malaria. The monk then planted some in his garden, just in case he should need them in the future.

After successfully treating his own illness, the monk became a doctor of some sort, and many malaria patients began coming to him for help. The monk treated them one by one, always with the roots of the same plant and always with the same good results. As time went on, people began to ask about the name of the plant. As it had no name, the monk began to tell his patients it was called "Mount Eternity."

Chinese: *Changshan* (Mount Eternity).

Re: 4321.
Common name: antipyretic dichroa.
Family: Saxifragaceae.
Chinese name: eternal mountain.
Scientific name: Dichroa febrifuga Lour.
Pharmaceutical name: Radix Dichroae.
Part used: root.
Dosage: 6 to 10 g.
Flavor: bitter.
Energy: cold.
Classes: herbs to expel or destroy parasites (class 18) and herbs to induce vomiting (class 7).
Meridians: lungs, heart, and liver.

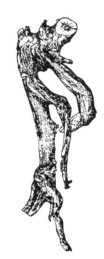

Actions: to induce vomiting of sputum, clear up heat, and promote water flow.

Indications: sputum, malaria, and amebic dysentery.

Notes: Experiments have shown *changshan* to be effective in treating various types of cancer, but it is slightly toxic, and should be consumed by pregnant women with great care. Before decoction, *changshan* must be fried in wine in order to reduce its side effect of nausea.

In Chinese herbalism, antipyretic dichroa is called Mount Eternity because the plants are so plentiful on that mountain. This plant has been used as an effective herb in treating malaria for many centuries. According to a report published in *Science,* antipyretic dichroa contains dichroine B, which has been proven effective for malaria. In another report, published in *Scientific Technology*, antipyretic dichroa was found to contain five different kinds of alkaloid, all of which are antimalarial agents, and one of them has been found to be five times more effective than quinine in treating malaria. The leaves, stalks, and roots are all effective, but the leaves have been found to be 20 times more effective than the roots, although the quantity of alkaloid contained in the leaves varies significantly from season to season.

A report published in the *Chinese Medical Journal* said that among the 24 cases of malaria treated by antipyretic dichroa, body temperature returned to normal within one day in 70 percent of the patients, and malarial parasites disappeared within two days in 50 percent of the patients. The treatment takes effect more slowly when three to four dosages are used daily, and takes effect more quickly when four to six dosages are used daily.

ASIAN DANDELION (FISHERMAN'S HERB, *PUGONGYING*)

The 16-year-old daughter of a government official in ancient China was suffering from mastitis with a triangular lump underneath her left breast. She was in pain and was becoming very worried, but she dared not tell anybody about it, because deep down inside she felt very ashamed. But her disease was subsequently found out by her maid, who disclosed it to her father, pleading with him to hire a doctor.

On inquiry into his daughter's condition, the official became very angry, as he suspected that his daughter must have done something immoral to have caused it. He rushed to his daughter's room and began to strike her in the face. "How could you do such a shameful thing, you are a disgrace to your family," shouted the father. The maid insisted that his daughter had never gone out alone and could not have possibly done anything immoral. The father wouldn't listen, and so the daughter ran away from home that night out of shame and desperation.

She went to the river bank, and, thinking that no one would be around at that hour to see her, quickly jumped into the river in an attempt to commit suicide. However, a fisherman was fishing from a rowboat nearby with his 16-year-old daughter. When they heard the splash, the fisherman's daughter instantly jumped into the river to save her. Once they were both on board, the fisherman was surprised to see that the girl was just about the same age as his daughter.

The fisherman's daughter began to change the girl's clothes, and in the process, discovered the swelling in the young lady's left breast. At that moment, she immediately understood the reason for her attempted suicide. After telling her father about it, the fisherman replied, "We will go dig some plants for her breast first thing in the morning."

72

The plant turned out to be a perennial herb, with white milky juice in it, yellowish flowers, and straight but fleshy and thick roots. They found the plants on the roadside not far from the river. They dug out a few plants that were about 100 g in weight, washed them clean, and boiled them in water. Then they told the girl to drink the liquid. In the meantime, they crushed some of the plants and applied them to her breast externally.

Upon hearing of the whereabouts and the attempted suicide of their daughter, the official and his wife, feeling greatly worried and deeply regretful, rushed to see the fisherman and to take their daughter home. Their daughter, grateful and in tears, said good-bye to the fisherman and his daughter and went home with her parents, bringing a bunch of the plants with her. Before she left, the fisherman kept reminding her to continue using the herbs for her illness.

After she had recovered from her illness, she told her maid to plant the herb in their garden. So that she would always remember the fisherman, she named the plant after him without knowing his name.

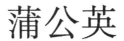

Chinese: *Pugongying* (Fisherman's Herb). **Re:** 5130.
Common name: Asian dandelion.
Family: Compositae.
Chinese name: yellow-flowered one-leg herb (so named because its flowers are yellow and the plant looks as if it has only one leg).
Scientific name: Taraxacum mongolicum Hand.-Mazz., Taraxacum sinicum Kitag., and Taraxacum heterolepis olepis Nakai et H. Koidz.
Pharmaceutical name: Herba Taraxaci.
Part used: entire plant.
Dosage: 20 g.
Flavor: bitter and sweet.
Energy: cold.
Class: 2, herbs to reduce excessive heat inside the body.
Meridians: spleen and stomach.

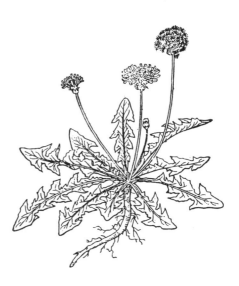

Actions: to clear up heat, counteract toxic effects, disperse swelling, and heal carbuncles.

Indications: carbuncles, swelling, mastitis, urinary infections, and acute tonsillitis.

Notes: Experts have shown that *pugongying* can be used for breast cancer, and that it is an antibacterial herb. It contains folic acid and bacterides, and it is now being widely used to treat mastitis, hepatitis, appendicitis, uri-

73

nary infections, acute tonsillitis, tracheitis, laryngitis, and the common cold.

In addition, *pugongying* can also regulate the liver and the stomach, which is why it can be used to treat mastitis and stomachache.

Asian dandelion is now used to treat many inflammatory diseases, including mumps, tonsillitis, and mastitis. Although this herb tastes bitter, the Chinese in the rural areas are in the habit of making tea out of it and then drinking it as a remedy for eye diseases, redness in the eyes, nose diseases, and urination disturbances.

The Chinese use Asian dandelion to treat such symptoms by decocting 50 g dandelion in two glasses of water until the water is reduced by half; then they strain it and drink the liquid once daily. In the treatment of eye disorders, they also take a cotton ball soaked in the fluid and press it over the closed eyes for about a half hour daily. Unlike most Chinese herbs, when Asian dandelion is used to treat inflammatory diseases, both internal and external methods should be applied, whether in treating mastitis, tonsillitis, or mumps.

According to a report published in *New Chinese Medicine,* Asian dandelion is effective for (1) indigestion and chronic constipation, (2) mastitis prior to pustulation by both internal and external applications simultaneously, (3) early stages of snake and insect bites prior to pustulation, and (4) promoting urination in treating acute urination disturbances, by the decoction of as much as 35 to 70 g of fresh dandelion, with smaller quantities producing little or no effect. The same report also indicated that when Asian dandelion is used as a tonic for the stomach, 10 to 20 g should be used for a one-day dosage by decoction, but when it is used to treat inflammatory diseases and to reduce swelling, 20 to 30 g should be used.

ASIATIC PLANTAIN (PLANT-BEFORE-CART, *CHEQIAN*) AND ASIATIC PLANTAIN SEED (SEED-BEFORE-CART, *CHEQIANZI*)

There was a Chinese general in the Han Dynasty (206 B.C.–A.D. 220) by the name of Ma-Wu. One summer, the country was undergoing a severe drought and the people were suffering from famine. As if things weren't bad enough for Ma-Wu, he had been defeated on the battlefield that summer and his entire army was forced to retreat to a remote region where nobody lived. Ma-Wu's soldiers couldn't find any water to drink there, nor could they find any food to eat. Many soldiers and horses died of starvation, and the surviving soldiers and horses had become so weak that virtually all of them had been under the attack of one disease or another. There was one particular symptom that almost every sick soldier and horse seemed to have—and that was presence of blood in the urine.

One of the grooms under Ma-Wu was in charge of three horses and one

74

cart. When this particular groom, who took his duties very seriously, saw that he and his three horses all showed blood in their urine, he desperately began to look for treatment.

One day, to his delight, the groom noticed that none of his three horses showed blood in their urine. Wondering what they possibly could have done, he made it a point to watch his horses very closely over the next few days, and noticed that they were eating plants that were a few inches tall and crept along the ground and had oblong leaves and light-green flowers. So, he pulled out a few plants, boiled them in water, and drank the liquid himself. After a few days of consuming this drink, the groom saw that the blood in his urine had completely disappeared.

The groom was so excited that he immediately told General Ma-Wu, who issued an order to all his soldiers to take this remedy themselves and to feed it to their horses. A few days later, none of the soldiers and their horses showed any sign of blood in their urine.

"Where did you find the plants?" the general asked the groom.

"I found them before the cart," replied the groom.

"What a wonderful plant before the cart!" shouted the general.

And so, the plant has been called "plant-before-cart" ever since.

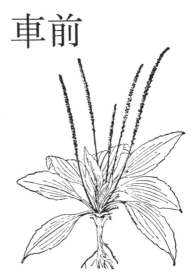

車前

Chinese: *Cheqian* (Plant-Before-Cart).
Re: 0799.
Common name: Asiatic plantain.
Family: Plantaginaceae.
Chinese name: before-the-cart grass.
Scientific names: Plantago asiatica L. and Plantago depressa Willd.
Pharmaceutical name: Herba Plantaginis.
Part used: entire plant.
Dosage: 10 to 18 g.
Flavor: sweet.
Energy: cold.
Class: 5, herbs to reduce dampness in the body.
Meridians: liver, spleen, and bladder.

Actions: to benefit water, clear heat, sharpen vision, and expel sputum.

Indications: chronic tracheitis, urination difficulty, vaginal discharge, blood in the urine, jaundice, edema, hot dysentery and diarrhea, nosebleed, pinkeye, eye pain, sore throat, cough, and skin ulcers.

Notes: Experiments indicate that this herb can benefit dampness and bring down blood pressure, as well as reduce blood fat and promote urination. However, this herb should be avoided by men with seminal emission due to kidney deficiency.

In Chinese herbalism, Asiatic plantain is called "plant before cart" because it can be found growing on the roadside along cart tracks. Both the seeds and leaves of Asiatic plantain are used as an herb and they have similar functions; however, the seeds are more commonly used than the leaves. One important use of this plant is to eliminate blood in the urine, as revealed in the legend, particularly in hot summer, when people have a tendency to develop urination disorders. Blood in the urine is frequently associated with difficulty in passing urine, and this plant can promote urination, which is why it is effective for this symptom.

Cheqian and *cheqianzi*, which is the seeds of this herb, are similar in certain effects, but *cheqian* can also clear heat and detoxicate, as well as clear the lungs and transform sputum. *Cheqian* is also good for skin eruptions and for cough due to lung heat. In addition, fresh *cheqian* can be used to treat diarrhea due to damp heat.

Chinese: *Cheqianzi* (Seed-Before-Cart).
Re: 0801.
Common name: Asiatic plantain seed.
Family: Plantaginaceae.
Chinese name: seed-before-cart.
Scientific names: Plantago asiatica L. and Plantago depressa Willd.
Pharmaceutical name: Semen Plantaginis.
Part used: ripe seed.
Dosage: 10 g.
Flavor: sweet.
Energy: cold.
Class: 5, herbs to reduce dampness in the body.
Meridians: liver, kidneys, and small intestine.

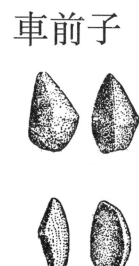

車前子

Actions: to clear up heat, benefit water, relieve cough, and expel sputum.
Indications: urination difficulty, edema, diarrhea, jaundice, and cough.
Notes: Experiments indicate that this herb is effective for suppression of cough and for promoting urination. Since the seeds are very small, they should be put in a cloth bag for decoction or they can be ground into powder for consumption.

76

BLACK FALSE HELLEBORE
(INSANITY GRASS, *LILU*)

Black false hellebore is a toxic herb, which even a goat or a cow will not eat. But how did this plant become an herb for curing diseases since it's so toxic?

As the story goes, a child by the name of Lilu suffered from epilepsy, and during a seizure, he would often become so violent that he would harm other children in the neighborhood. In fact, one time he hurt a child so severely that his parents were forced to pay a large sum of money in compensation.

One day Lilu's parents and his brothers were talking about the situation with Lilu, and the oldest son said, "What if Lilu kills someone the next time? If that happens, the whole family would suffer terribly."

"I agree," said another brother, "so why don't we put Lilu to death?" Lilu's parents felt terrible about the thought of putting him to death, but since they couldn't figure out a better solution, they remained silent.

The following day, Lilu was undergoing another epileptic seizure. Anticipating the possibility of violence, Lilu's oldest brother pushed him to the ground and forced a cup of fresh black false hellebore juice into his mouth, in an attempt to poison him to death. Lilu began to vomit a few minutes later. His brother then forced another cup of the juice into his mouth, and Lilu began to vomit again. When Lilu finally stopped vomiting, he got up and walked into the kitchen to eat a bowl of rice. From that point on, Lilu never had another seizure. This herb was appropriately named after Lilu.

Chinese: *Lilu* (Insanity Grass).
Re: 5652.
Common name: black false hellebore.
Family: Liliaceae.
Chinese name: black false hellebore.
Scientific name: Veratrum nigrum L.
Pharmaceutical name: Rhizoma et Radix Veratri Nigri.
Part used: rhizome.
Dosage: 1 to 1.5 g.
Flavor: bitter and pungent.
Energy: cold.
Class: 7, herbs to induce vomiting.
Meridians: liver, lungs, and stomach.
Actions: to induce vomiting of undigested foods and sputum, and destroy worms.
Indications: epilepsy, accumulation of sputum, indigestion, and scabies (by external application).

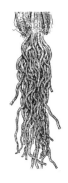

Notes: Lilu is a strong emetic (vomitive) and can also drive out wind sputum in excess diseases and destroy worms; but since it is toxic, it should not be used by pregnant women and those with deficiency and loss of blood.

BONESET (SISTER-IN-LAW'S ORCHID, *PEILAN*) AND KOREAN MINT (SISTER-IN-LAW'S MINT, *HUOXIANG*)

Once upon a time, a young couple and the husband's sister were living together in a small village. After the husband went off to join the army, his wife and sister remained living together. The wife was named Peilan and the sister Huoxiang, and the two were very nice to each other and lived in harmony.

One summer Peilan suffered a sunstroke with a headache, dizziness, palpitations, and nausea. Huoxiang put her in bed, telling her, "My brother taught me how to use two herbs to cure sunstroke. Let me go pick them in the mountains and decoct them for you to drink."

Peilan protested, saying that the mountains were too dangerous, but Huoxiang insisted on going anyway.

Peilan stayed in bed, waiting for Huoxiang to come back, but she did not return until early the next morning. No sooner had Huoxiang entered Peilan's bedroom, than she fainted and fell to the floor.

"What happened, Huoxiang?" asked Peilan, once Huoxiang had regained consciousness.

"I've been bitten by a poisonous snake," replied Huoxiang.

Realizing that snake bites could be fatal, Peilan tried to suck the poison from Huoxiang's wound. But it was all in vain; Huoxiang died an hour later. A neighbor who suspected something strange going on came knocking at the door, but nobody answered. So, the neighbor came in anyway and was astonished to see both Peilan and Huoxiang lying on the floor. Huoxiang was already dead, and Peilan was on the verge of death.

Peilan explained, "Huoxiang went to the mountains to dig up two herbs for me—one for vomiting and diarrhea, and one for vomiting and dizziness, particularly in the summer. Please remember these two herbs, just in case someone needs them."

No sooner had Peilan finished her last word, than she died.

Afterwards, the neighbor named the two herbs after Peilan and Huoxiang.

Chinese: *Peilan* (Sister-in-Law's Orchid). 佩羌
Re: 2841.
Common name: boneset.

78

Family: Compositae.

Chinese name: wearing orchid (so named because when it's worn, this herb smells like an orchid).

Scientific names: Eupatorium fortunei Turcz. and japonicum Thunberg.

Pharmaceutical name: Herba Eupatorii.

Parts used: stalks and leaves.

Dosage: 8 g.

Flavor: pungent.

Energy: neutral.

Class: 5, herbs to reduce dampness in the body.

Meridians: lungs and spleen.

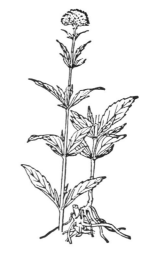

Actions: to transform dampness by aromatic flavor, and relieve summer heat.

Indications: Headache due to summer heat.

Notes: *Peilan* has a very strong aroma and can transform dampness and clear summer heat rather effectively. Experiments have shown that *peilan* can inhibit influenza.

Huoxiang and *peilan* can be decocted together to harmonize the stomach and relieve vomiting. This formula is good for vomiting and abdominal swelling due to summer heat.

Chinese: *Huoxiang* (Sister-in-Law's Mint).

Re: 5685.

Common name: Korean mint.

Family: Labiatae.

Chinese name: aromatic bean leaf (so named because the leaves of this herb look like those of a bean, and it smells aromatic).

Scientific names: Agastache rugosus (Fisch. et Mey) O. Ktze. and Pogostemon cablin (Blanco) Benth.

Pharmaceutical name: Herba Agastchis.

Part used: stalk leaves.

Dosage: 8 g.

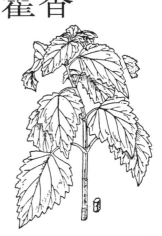

79

Flavor: pungent.

Energy: slightly warm.

Class: 5, herbs to reduce dampness in the body (specifically those herbs that transform dampness by their aromatic smell).

Meridians: spleen and stomach.

Actions: to transform dampness, harmonize the stomach, and relieve vomiting.

Indications: Nausea and vomiting.

Notes: *Huoxiang* is pungent, warm, and aromatic, and it can stimulate the spleen, regulate the stomach, warm the middle region, transform dampness, relieve stomach stagnation, and relieve vomiting. Experiments have shown that *huoxiang* is effective as a digestive, and that it can inhibit influenza and also relieve vomiting.

CARRIZO (REED RHIZOME, *LUGEN*)

There was a small village in southern China with only one herb shop, and the owner kept raising his prices. One day a child from a poor family suffered high fever, so the child's mother went to the shop to get some herbs. The owner of the shop told her that her child needed antelope's horn, which was a very expensive animal product, but the mother couldn't afford it. When she asked the shopkeeper if he would sell it to her at a cheaper price, he refused her.

So the mother went home empty-handed, and her child's fever continued. Later that day a beggar knocked at her door and asked for a bowl of rice.

"We are a poor family, and this is the only bowl of rice left," said the mother, as she handed it to him, with tears in her eyes.

"What is wrong, Ma'am? Why are you crying?" inquired the beggar.

The mother told him that her child had a high fever and she couldn't afford to buy antelope's horn.

"You don't need antelope's horn for high fever," said the beggar. "Those plants growing near the pond will work just as well."

On the advice of the beggar, the mother picked the plants and decocted them for her child to drink, which quickly reduced the fever, and the child recovered completely a short time later. The plants she picked were *lugen.*

Chinese: *Lugen* (Reed Rhizome).　　蘆根
Re: 2191.
Common name: reed rhizome.

80

Family: Gramineae.
Chinese name: Reed rhizome.
Scientific name: Phragmites communis (L.) Trin.
Pharmaceutical name: Rhizoma Phragmitis.
Part used: rhizome.
Dosage: 20 g.
Flavor: sweet.
Energy: cold.
Class: 2, herbs to reduce excessive heat inside the body.
Meridians: lungs, stomach, and kidneys.

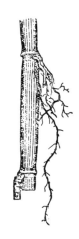

Actions: to clear up heat, produce fluids, and promote urination.
Indications: thirst, short stream of urine, vomiting due to a hot stomach, dry cough due to hot lungs, and lung disease.
Notes: *Lugen* can clear heat, produce fluids, and quench thirst.

CHEROKEE ROSE (GOLDEN-TASSEL SEED, *JINYINGZI*)

Once upon a time, there were three brothers who lived together with their wives. But only one of the couples had a child, and this child grew up as the only child in this big family. After some time, all the members of the family were very anxious to see this only son in the family get married and have children. But no girl would marry him because he had a problem—bed-wetting. And so the family tried to find a cure for it.

One day an old herbalist, carrying a bag with a golden tassel, came to the village to sell some herbs. One of the brothers asked the herbalist if he had any herbs in his bag that could cure bed-wetting. The herbalist said he didn't but that he knew of one herb that could cure it that could be found in southern China. He further explained that since it would require a long journey to travel there to get the herb, they would have to pay him a huge sum of money. However, the family agreed and the old herbalist undertook the journey.

Many months passed, but the old herbalist did not return, and the family had virtually given up hope, when one evening there was a knock at their door. One of the brothers opened the door and was astonished to see the old herbalist, who had fainted beside the door. He immediately carried the old herbalist into the house. Once he regained consciousness, the herbalist told the family that the herb he got in southern China was in his bag, but his voice was so low that the family could hardly hear him. The herbalist died a few days later due to physical exhaustion.

81

Nevertheless, the family decocted the herb, which successfully cured their son's bed-wetting. They did not know the name of the herb nor did they know the name of the old herbalist, so they decided to call the herb "golden-tassel seed," after the golden tassel attached to the old man's bag and because the seed of the plant is used as the herb.

Chinese: *Jinyingzi* (Golden-Tassel Seed).
Re: 2898.

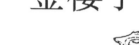

Common name: Japanese honey-suckle.
Family: Rosaceae.
Chinese name: golden-cherry seed.
Scientific name: Rosa laevigata Michx.
Pharmaceutical name: Fructus Rosae Laevigatae.
Part used: ripe fruit.
Dosage: 7 to 15 g.
Flavor: sweet and sour.
Energy: neutral.
Class: 17, herbs to constrict and obstruct movements.
Meridians: kidneys, spleen, and lungs.

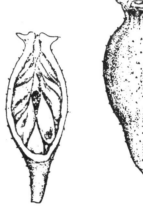

Actions: to benefit the kidneys, constrict semen, and relieve diarrhea.
Indications: frequent urination, enuresis, chronic diarrhea, seminal emission, and vaginal bleeding and discharge.
Notes: Experiments have shown *jinyingzi* to be effective as a digestive, in inhibiting gastrointestinal peristalsis, and in stopping diarrhea. *Jinyingzi* is obstructive and should be avoided by those with constipation.

Jinyingzi can be decocted with *qianshi* (chicken head kernel) to solidify semen and check urination. This combination is especially beneficial for frequent urination due to kidney deficiency.

CHINESE CLEMATIS (TEMPLE'S HOLY ROOT, *WEILINGXIAN*)

At the top of a high mountain in southern China, there was a temple called "the temple of powerful spirits," which was managed by an old nun who was also a knowledgeable herbalist. She used herbs to treat the illnesses of the people who came to worship at the temple, most of whom suffered from rheumatism and arthritis.

The old nun-herbalist was a very cunning person, and did not want to let people know that she was treating them with herbs. Instead, she would give a patient a cup of soup, explaining that it was the soup of Buddha, which could cure diseases because of its powerful spirits, and the patient

82

would believe her. The old nun did this in an attempt to get more people to worship at the temple and to collect more donations.

A young nun who was working under the old nun knew about her secret, because it was she who decocted the herbs for the patients. This young nun was often mistreated by the old nun, and she was very unhappy about it. On top of that, she felt it was wrong for the old nun to deceive people into thinking that it was the powerful spirits of Buddha that cured their diseases, and not the healing power of herbs.

One day, when the young nun was told by the old nun to decoct an herb for a patient, she deliberately decocted a different herb. The patient drank it and of course did not improve. Day after day, the same thing happened, and many people even found their illnesses getting worse. After a while, people stopped coming to see the old nun, and went to see the young nun instead.

One day, when the old nun found out that people were going to the young nun for treatment, she went into a frenzy and died from a heart attack. The young nun took over the temple and gave people free treatments. The herb that she used to treat their arthritis and rheumatism had no name, so the young nun named it "temple's holy root."

Chinese: *Weilingxian* (Temple's Holy Root). 威靈仙

Re: 3372.

Common name: Chinese clematis.

Family: Ranunculaceae.

Chinese name: powerful soul root.

Scientific names: Clematis chinensis Osbeck, Clematis hexapetala Pall., and Clematis manshurica Rupr.

Pharmaceutical name: Radix Clematidis.

Part used: root.

Dosage: 3 to 10 g.

Flavor: pungent.

Energy: warm.

Class: 3, herbs to counteract rheumatism.

Meridian: bladder.

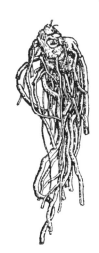

Actions: to remove wind and dampness, facilitate passage of meridians, and relieve pain.

Indications: rheumatism, jaundice, and edema.

Notes: *Weilingxian* is an effective herb for treating wind-cold rheumatism. Experiments have shown that *weilingxian* can benefit the gallbladder and reduce jaundice, and that it is also an effective herb for relief of pain and rheumatism.

83

CHINESE EPHEDRAA (ASK-FOR-TROUBLE, *MAHUANG*)

A Chinese herbalist with no son decided to accept a disciple to help him with his work, and to whom he could teach his trade. The disciple was an impatient person, and after having studied under his master for only a few months, wanted to open a clinic of his own. However, the old herbalist was reluctant to let him go, not merely because he needed his help but because he didn't think he was ready for his own patients.

"Before you leave me to operate your own clinic, there is one thing you should remember," warned the old herbalist. "There is a plant whose leaves and roots have opposite effects: The leaves can induce perspiration, whereas the roots can reduce it. You must keep this in mind in treating your patients."

But the disciple was caught up in his own plans, and barely heard what his master was saying.

On the grand-opening day of the clinic, the son of a judge fell ill and was perspiring profusely, so the judge brought his son to the clinic. The former disciple used the leaves of a plant to treat the young patient, and he used the herb in huge amounts, intending to produce quick results. Rather unexpectedly, the patient began to perspire even more profusely after taking the herb. And his arms and legs became as cold as ice; in fact, his entire body was shivering with cold.

The judge was furious and rushed his son to the old herbalist, who then told the judge that his former disciple had used the wrong part of the plant; instead of using the roots of the plant, he had used the leaves, without realizing that the leaves could actually induce perspiration.

The judge later summoned the young herbalist, and told him, "In treating patients without much knowledge, you are asking for trouble." Hence, the plant came to be known as "ask-for-trouble."

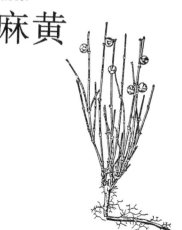

Chinese: *Mahuang* (Ask-For-Trouble). 麻黄
Re: 4615.
Common name: Chinese ephedra.
Family: Ephedraceae.
Chinese name: numb yellow herb (so named because it produces numb sensations and is yellow).
Scientific names: Ephedra sinica Stapf, Ephedra intermedia Schrenk et C. A. May, and Ephedra equisetina Bge.
Pharmaceutical name: Herba Ephedrae.

84

Part used: dry stalks.
Dosage: 6 g.
Flavor: pungent and bitter.
Energy: warm.
Class: 1, herbs to induce perspiration.
Meridians: lungs and bladder.

Actions: to induce perspiration; to disperse cold (when raw), overcome asthma (when fried), and promote urination.

Indications: asthma, edema, and hypertension (if used with great care).

Notes: *Mahuang* can be decocted with *kuxingren* (bitter apricot) to reinforce the effect of calming asthma.

Experiments have shown that *mahuang* is effective for asthma, and can promote urination and inhibit influenza. *Mahuang* contains ephedrine, which accounts for its effectiveness in treating asthma.

In the treatment of asthma, *mahuang* should be used intermittently, particularly in chronic asthma, because a continuous, prolonged use of it can decrease its effects, as the patient may develop a resistance to it. In addition, *mahuang* can excite the cerebral cortex, which may lead to nervousness and insomnia.

When patients suffering from the common cold are perspiring profusely, *mahuang* should not be used for treatment, because *mahuang* is a relatively strong herb for inducing perspiration.

The following precautions should be taken in using *mahuang:* (1) Do not use excessive doses (normally between 1.5 and 10 g are recommended); (2) when *mahuang* is decocted with other herbs, it should be decocted first so that the floating bubbles can be removed from the water; and (3) those with deficient body energy and excessive perspiration should avoid *mahuang*.

Mahuanggen is the root of *mahuang* and produces opposing effects.

Chinese: *Mahuanggen* (Root of Chinese Ephedra).
Re: 4624.
Common name: Chinese ephedra root.
Family: Ephedraceae.
Chinese name: hemp yellow root.
Scientific names: Ephedra sinica Stapf and Ephedra intermedia Schrenk et C. A. Mey.
Pharmaceutical name: Radix Ephedrae.
Part used: root.
Dosage: 3 to 10 g.
Flavor: sweet.
Energy: neutral.

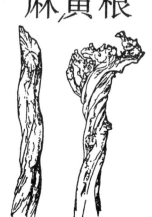

麻黄根

Class: 17, herbs to constrict and obstruct movements.
Meridians: lungs.
Actions: to check perspiration.
Indications: excessive perspiration and night sweats.

CHINESE GINSENG (MAN'S PLANT, *RENSHEN*) AND WESTERN GINSENG

There was an old hunter with two sons who were just learning how to hunt. Before they left to go hunting on their own for the first time, he advised them to wait until winter was over. But the two brothers insisted on going anyway.

Within a few days, they had killed quite a few animals. Then one afternoon the weather suddenly changed and snow began to fall, virtually blocking all the passages out of the mountains. One week later, they were still unable to get out of the mountains and they had run out of food. In desperation, they searched everywhere for something to eat.

They finally spotted a plant that looked different from the others. After digging it out of the ground, the two brothers were surprised to see that the roots resembled a man standing up. They began to eat the roots, which tasted sweet and a little bitter and were very juicy. They continued eating them over the next few days, and found that they were becoming very energetic. Thinking that in cold winter, they needed plenty of energy, they ate the roots in huge amounts, but then one of them began to develop a nosebleed. So, they decided to eat the roots in moderate amounts. The roots of this plant tided them over through the winter. And in spring, when the snow melted away, they headed home.

Meanwhile, the father of the two brothers was deeply worried, and the people in the village all thought that the brothers had died.

The unexpected return of the two brothers shocked the entire village. Of course, the old hunter was relieved that his sons were still alive, but he did not understand how they had managed to survive under such severe conditions.

"How did you make it through the cold winter in the mountains?" asked the father.

"We ate the roots of a plant," explained one of the brothers.

"What is the name of the plant?" asked the father.

"We don't know the name of the plant," said the other brother," but its roots look like a man."

"Oh! It must be man's plant," said the father.

86

Chinese: *Renshen* (Man's Plant).

Re: 0055.

Common name: ginseng.

Family: Araliaceae.

Chinese name: man's plant (so named because the roots of this plant resemble the shape of a man).

Scientific name: Panax ginseng C. A. Mey.

Pharmaceutical name: Radix Ginseng.

Part used: root.

Dosage: 5 g.

Flavor: sweet and slightly bitter.

Energy: warm.

Class: 16, herbs to correct deficiencies.

Meridians: spleen and lungs.

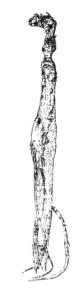

Actions: to tone up original energy drastically, fix prolapse, produce fluids, secure spirits, and benefit brain.

Indications: weakness after chronic illness, vaginal bleeding, diabetes, prolapse, palpitations, and forgetfulness.

Notes: Experiments have shown that *renshen* is an effective heart tonic and anti-shock herb. It can increase red blood cells and produce adrenocortical hormones, sex hormones, and excitation, as well as reduce blood sugar and blood fat.

There are three basic varieties of *renshen* (radix ginseng): wild ginseng, which is found in the mountains in the northeastern Chinese provinces, notably Jilin and Heilongjiang; red ginseng, which is cultivated ginseng that has been steamed to become red; and Korean ginseng, which is produced in Korea and processed with medicinal plants.

Wild ginseng tastes sweet and slightly bitter and warm. It is most frequently used as a single ingredient to drastically tonify energy, tonify the lungs and the spleen, benefit yin, produce fluids, and secure the spirits; it is also used as first-aid treatment for prolapse caused by severe bleeding. Red ginseng has the same properties as wild ginseng but is weaker in its effects, while Korean ginseng is warmer and can tonify yang more effectively.

Chinese ginseng (radix ginseng) can tonify energy more effectively than Western ginseng (radix panacis quinquefolii), which is why in treating symptoms of prolapse, Chinese ginseng can be applied all by itself. Western ginseng is cool in energy, and can produce fluids; it is most appropriate for patients with high fever and energy deficiency simultaneously.

87

Chinese: *Xiyangshen* (Western ginseng).
Re: 1713.
Common name: Western ginseng.
Family: Araliaceae.
Chinese name: Western ginseng.
Scientific name: Panax quinquefolium Linne.
Pharmaceutical name: Radix Panacis Quinquefolii.
Part used: root.
Dosage: 8 g.
Flavor: bitter and sweet.
Energy: cool.
Class: 16, herbs to correct deficiencies.
Meridians: lungs and stomach.
Actions: to tone up the lungs, benefit energy, nourish stomach, produce fluids, and clear up heat.
Indications: yin deficiency with internal heat, thirst, cough, and voice loss.

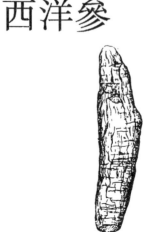

CHINESE HAWTHORN (MOUNTAIN HAWTHORN, *SHANZHA*)

A forty-year-old businessman was once married and had a son; two years after his wife died, he got married again to a cunning woman who disliked her stepchild and wanted to get rid of him.

"What is the best way to do it?" she pondered. "I can't kill him, nor can I poison him to death, because people will find out."

After her husband left on a business trip, she decided to take some action against her stepchild, who was almost ten years old. Her stepchild worked in the mountains every day, and she always brought him his lunch. While her husband was gone, she intentionally prepared his lunch with half-cooked rice, with the hope that he would die from indigestion. After a few weeks, the stepchild began to complain of indigestion and was starting to lose weight. This pleased the stepmother and she continued to make him lunch with half-cooked rice.

One day the stepchild happened to find a tree growing with plenty of berries. He picked some berries out of curiosity, and ate them and found them delicious. These berries seemed to quench his thirst as well. He began to feel better and continued to eat the berries every day, gradually putting on weight.

"What is happening to this child?" the stepmother asked herself. "He is not dying—on the contrary, he looks much healthier. . . . Maybe God is protecting this child."

88

Being fearful of God, the stepmother stopped making his lunch with half-cooked rice. When the businessman returned home, he learned about the berries from his son and decided to market them to herbalists in town.

Chinese: *Shanzha* (Mountain Hawthorn).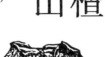
Re: 0323.
Common name: Chinese hawthorn.
Family: Rosaceae.
Chinese name: red fruits (so named because its fruits are red).
Scientific name: Crataegus pinnatifida Bge. var. major N.E.Br.
Pharmaceutical name: Fructus Crataegi.
Part used: fruit.
Dosage: 10 g.
Flavor: sour.
Energy: slightly warm.
Class: 9, herbs to promote digestion.
Meridians: spleen, stomach, and liver.

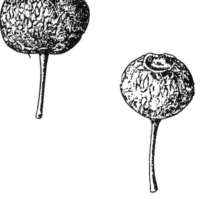

Actions: to eliminate accumulations, promote energy flow, and disperse coagulations.

Indications: indigestion, dysentery, hernia, blood coagulations, and suppression of menses.

Notes: According to experiments, *shanzha* is an effective heart tonic; it can activate the blood and bring down blood pressure, it is effective as a digestive, it can treat fatty liver, and it can also reduce blood fat.

Shanzha is a strong herb for transforming food and eliminating food stagnation due to indigestion; it is particularly effective for eliminating meat indigestion.

Shanzha can activate the blood and remove blood coagulations. It is often used in conjunction with *danggui* and *yimucao* to treat pain in the lower abdomen and lochiostasis.

CHINESE PULSATILLA (GRANDPA'S GREY HAIR, *BAITOUWENG*)

A young man suffered from abdominal pain with diarrhea, which made him perspire profusely. He went to see a doctor, but the doctor wasn't in, so the young man had no choice but to return home. On his way home, his abdominal pain became so severe that he had to lie down on the wayside to rest.

89

An old man with grey hair all over his head walked up to him and said, "Young man, what is wrong with you? Why are you lying here?"

"I am having unbearable abdominal pain," the young man replied.

"Why don't you see a doctor?" asked the old man.

"I went to see a doctor, but the doctor wasn't there," explained the young man.

Then an idea dawned on the old man. "You don't need a doctor," he said. "The plant beside you is a good remedy for abdominal pain and diarrhea. Pick some and decoct the roots. I promise it will relieve your suffering."

The young man looked at the old man in disbelief, but he picked some plants anyway and started for home after his abdominal pain had somewhat subsided.

Soon after he got home, his pain started again with severe diarrhea. Thinking that he had nothing to lose, the young man began to decoct the roots of the plant; he had the soup a few times, and shortly got relief from the symptoms.

Good news travels fast, and soon the whole village knew about it. People started to inquire about the plant, but all the young man could tell them was that an old man who was about the age of his grandpa with grey hair all over his head told him to use it. Thus, the herb came to be known as "grandpa's grey hair."

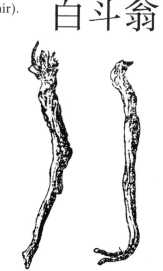

白斗翁

Chinese: *Baitouweng* (Grandpa's Grey Hair).
Re: 1411.
Common name: Chinese pulsatilla.
Family: Ranunculaceae.
Chinese name: white-headed man.
Scientific name: Pulsatilla chinensis (Bge.) Regel.
Pharmaceutical name: Radix Pulsatillae.
Part used: whole plant.
Dosage: 10 to 18 g.
Flavor: bitter.
Energy: cold.
Class: 2, herbs to reduce excessive heat inside the body.
Meridians: stomach and large intestine.

Actions: to clear up heat, detoxicate cool blood, and relieve dysentery.

Indications: dysentery, nosebleed, and hemorrhoids.

Notes: According to experiments, *baitouweng* is an effective heart tonic and can stop diarrhea.

90

CHINESE YAM (MOUNTAIN MEDICINE, *SHANYAO*)

Two kingdoms were at war with each other, with the stronger kingdom having won the last battle. All the soldiers in the defeated kingdom escaped to a high mountain to hide from their enemies, but they were soon surrounded by the victorious soldiers, with their lines of communication completely cut off. Thinking that the soldiers on the mountain would have no choice but to surrender sooner or later, or else starve to death, the victorious army began to enjoy themselves at the foot of the mountain. Having surrounded them for a full year, strangely enough they had not seen a single surrendering enemy soldier come down from the mountain. Then one night a strong army of soldiers suddenly appeared from the mountain to break the encirclement below and scored a decisive victory over the stronger kingdom.

What had the soldiers eaten on the mountain? After their food supply had run out, they started looking for something to eat, and found plenty of plants with big roots, which they ate as food while their horses ate the vines of the plants. Since the plants were growing on the mountain and their roots were as powerful as medicine, the soldiers called the plants "mountain medicine."

Chinese: *Shanyao* (Mountain Medicine).
Re: 0319.
Common name: Chinese yam.
Family: Dioscoreaceae.
Chinese name: mountain medicine.
Scientific names: Dioscorea opposita Thunb. and Dioscorea batatas Decaisne.
Pharmaceutical names: Rhizoma Dioscoreae and Rhizoma Batatatis.
Part used: tuberous root.
Dosage: 15 g.
Flavor: sweet.
Energy: neutral.
Class: 16, herbs to correct deficiencies.
Meridians: spleen, stomach, lungs, and kidneys.

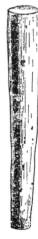

Actions: to strengthen the spleen and stomach, relieve diarrhea, and tone up the lungs and kidneys.
Indications: spleen deficiency with poor appetite, chronic diarrhea, seminal emission, vaginal discharge, and diabetes.

91

Notes: According to experiments, *shanyao* can reduce blood sugar. It can also tonify the spleen and stop diarrhea, particularly diarrhea due to spleen deficiency, and vaginal discharge in women.

COIN GRASS (*JINQIANCAO*)

A loving couple was living happily in a small village, but since nothing lasts forever, one day the husband developed a pain below his ribs, as if he were being cut by a knife, and died a few days later. The wife was so saddened and so puzzled by her husband's sudden death that she insisted on having an autopsy conducted. A stone was found in her husband's gallbladder. The wife took the stone with her, but was still perplexed by how a single stone could have killed her husband. She hung this stone in front of her neck on a string, however, and kept it there day and night for many years.

One autumn, she went to the mountains to cut some plants, which she carried back home by hand. By the time she got home, she was surprised to find that the size of the stone in front of her neck had shrunk by half. She told everyone she knew about the incident, but no one seemed to believe her. Then one day an herbalist heard about it and became very curious.

"What kind of plants did you bring home that day? Could you take me to the place where you picked them?" he asked her.

The woman took the herbalist to the mountains where she picked the plants, but all the plants were gone. The two had no choice but to wait until the next year.

In the autumn of the following year, the woman and the herbalist went to the mountains once again. They cut the plants and the woman brought them home in the same manner as she had the previous year. But this time, the stone remained the same size.

In the autumn of the third year, the two went to the same place again. They cut different kinds of plants and put the stone on each of them for a period of time, finally coming upon a plant that dissolved the stone.

"This is a great discovery indeed!" exclaimed the herbalist. "We have found a cure for stones in the gallbladder."

Chinese: *Jinqiancao* (Coin Grass).　　金錢草
Re: 2889.
Common name: herb of longtube ground ivy.
Family: Labiatae.

92

Chinese name: golden coin grass (so named because the leaves of the plant are as round as a coin).
Scientific name: Glechoma longituba (Nakai) Kupr.
Pharmaceutical name: Herba Glechoma.
Part used: whole plant.
Dosage: 15 to 25 g.
Flavor: bitter and pungent.
Energy: cool.
Class: 5, herbs to reduce dampness in the body.
Meridians: undetermined.

Actions: to clear up heat, promote urination, suppress cough, heal swelling, and counteract toxic effects.

Indications: jaundice, edema, gallstones, malaria, lung disease, cough, vomiting of blood, and rheumatism.

Notes: Experiments have shown that *jinqiancao* can (1) benefit the gallbladder and reduce jaundice, (2) promote liver bile production and bile excretion, (3) expel hepatic calculus (hepatolith), (4) expel urinary stones, (5) be used as an adjuvant herb to treat liver and gallbladder diseases, and (6) promote urination.

DANGGUI (OUGHT-TO-RETURN)

A high mountain in China was full of precious herbs, but few people climbed it to pick them because the route was so treacherous.

One day a group of young men were talking among themselves and one fellow boasted, "I am the bravest of us all."

"If you're so brave," said another fellow, "I dare you to climb that mountain and bring back some herbs."

"I accept your challenge!" declared the young man.

When he told his mother of his intention to climb the mountain, she strongly objected at first, but then later relented, saying "You are my only son, and I will be completely alone after you are gone. Since you are already engaged, why don't you at least get married before you go, so that I will not be alone?"

The young man agreed and got married. Before he left, he told his wife to remarry should he fail to return home in three years, as the route through the mountain was so hazardous.

The young man did not return in one year, nor did he return in two years, nor in three years. So, the young man's mother told her daughter-

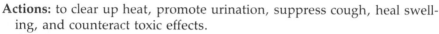

93

in-law to remarry. She hesitated at first but then agreed, thinking that her husband must have died on the mountain.

However, a few days after her marriage, the young man suddenly returned home, which shocked everyone in the small village. All of his friends praised him for his great courage in climbing the mountain and thanked him for the many precious herbs he had picked and brought home. In the midst of the excitement, the young man was puzzled by the absence of his wife. After inquiring as to her whereabouts, he was told that she had just remarried.

Regretting his failure to return within three years, the young man asked to meet with his former wife. But on hearing of her former husband's return, the wife had burst into tears and had become seriously ill. One of the herbs the young man had picked on the mountain was a great tonic for women, so he decocted the herb and gave it to her to drink, and it cured her illness in a few days.

To commemorate this incident, a Chinese poet wrote, "He ought to return a little sooner but failed to return; she ought to wait a little longer but failed to wait." The herb was thus named "ought-to-return."

Chinese: *Dangreg* (Ought-to-Return).

當歸

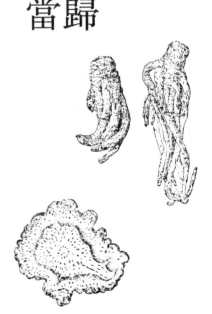

Re: 1763.

Common name: *Dangreg.*

Family: Umbelliferae.

Chinese name: ought-to-return (so named because, according to Chinese herbalogy, by taking this herb, one's energy and blood will return without disorder).

Scientific name: Angelica sinensis (Oliv.) Diels.

Pharmaceutical name: Radix Angelicae Sinensis.

Part used: root.

Dosage: 10 g.

Flavor: sweet and pungent.

Energy: warm.

Class: 16, herbs to correct deficiencies.

Meridians: heart, liver, and spleen.

Actions: to tone up blood, activate blood, regulate menstruation, and produce intestinal sliding.

Indications: blood deficiency and coagulation causing suppression of menses and abdominal pain; rheumatism and constipation.

94

Notes: Experiments have shown that *danggui* can protect the liver and regulate menstruation, and that it contains volatile oils and folic acid.

Since *danggui* can tonify and activate the blood simultaneously, it is an effective herb for women. *Danggui* and *shudihuang* are two of the most important blood tonics.

DODDER (BUNNY'S SEED, *TUSIZI*)

A young man was hired by a farmer to look after his bunnies. Being a harsh taskmaster, the farmer warned the young man that the death of a bunny would cost him a quarter of his wages, which made the young man very nervous.

One day this young man accidentally dropped a bamboo stick on a bunny, which broke her spine; the bunny lay on the ground unable to move. The young man was afraid that his boss would find out, so he took the bunny from the pen and hid her in the field of soybean plants, where the poor bunny lay very still as if dying.

The farmer found one bunny missing, so the young man went to the field to bring the bunny back. To his surprise, the bunny was running around in the field. He chased after the bunny for quite a while, before finally catching her and bringing her back to the pen.

Then the young man intentionally broke another bunny's back and brought her to the soybean field. A few days later, he saw that the bunny's back had completely healed.

"How could that have happened?" he later asked his father, who suffered from a backache and had laid in bed for many years.

"Maybe it's the soybean plants," mused his father.

The next day, the young man deliberately broke the back of yet another bunny and brought her to the field. But this time, he watched closely what the bunny ate. He found that the bunny was not eating the soybean plants at all, but rather the seeds of a parasitic plant living on them. A few days later, the bunny had recovered from her back injury.

The young man started to pick the seeds of this parasitic plant and then decocted them for his father to drink; soon afterwards, his father's backache was cured! The herb has been known as "bunny's seed" ever since.

Chinese: *Tusizi* (Bunny's Seed).
Re: 4125.
Common name: dodder seed.
Family: Convolvulaceae.
Chinese name: hare silk seed.
Scientific names: Cuscuta chinensis Lam. and Cuscuta japonica Choisy.
Pharmaceutical name: Semen Cuscutae.

Part used: ripe seed.
Dosage: 5 to 10 g.
Flavor: pungent and sweet.
Energy: neutral.
Class: 16, herbs to correct deficiencies.
Meridians: liver and kidneys.
Actions: to tone up the liver and the kidneys, strengthen yang, and relieve diarrhea.
Indications: impotence, seminal emission, diarrhea, lumbago, and insecure fetus.

Notes: *Tusizi* can tonify the liver and the kidneys to treat lumbago and weak legs due to liver and kidney deficiencies. It is an effective herb for the treatment of impotence, seminal emission, and premature ejaculation, and enuresis due to kidney deficiency.

EVERGREEN ARTEMISIA (EVERGREEN SPIRE, *YINCHENHAO*)

Once a fellow suffered from jaundice, with a yellowish complexion and depressed eyes. His friends called him "Mr. Cockroach," because he had lost so much weight that he looked like a cockroach.

One day Mr. Cockroach went to see a famous doctor named Hua Duo. But Dr. Hua Duo told him that there was no cure for jaundice, so Mr. Cockroach sadly returned home.

A few months later, when Dr. Hua Duo ran into Mr. Cockroach on the street, he was surprised to see him still alive and in good health. He asked him who had treated him and what he had taken, but was told that the jaundice had disappeared all by itself. Dr. Hua Duo could not believe it, so Mr. Cockroach further explained that due to his illness, he had run out of money over the past few months and had to live on one particular plant as food. He then took Dr. Hua Duo to see the plant, which Dr. Hua Duo subsequently started using to treat his jaundice patients. But to his disappointment, the treatments didn't work, which puzzled Dr. Hua Duo a great deal.

After questioning Mr. Cockroach, Dr. Hua Duo was convinced that he had in fact identified the right plant, which he had picked in March of the previous year. Thinking that the timing of picking the plant might have something to do with its effects, Dr. Hua Duo picked the plant that March and used it to treat his patients with jaundice, and this time all the patients recovered. Dr. Hua Duo then concluded that only the tender leaves and branches picked in March could be used to treat jaundice.

Chinese: *Yinchenhao* (Evergreen Spire).
Re: 3305.
Common name: herb of virgate wormwood and herb of capillary wormwood.
Family: Compositae.
Chinese name: mattress old wormwood.
Scientific name: Artemisia capillaris Thunberg.
Pharmaceutical names: Herba Artemisiae Capillaris and Herba Artemisiae Scopariae.
Parts used: seedlings and spires.
Dosage: 15 to 30 g.
Flavor: bitter and pungent.
Energy: slightly cold.
Class: 5, herbs to remove dampness in the body.
Meridian: bladder.

茵陳蒿

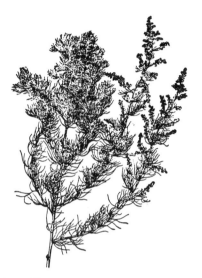

Actions: to clear up damp heat and reduce jaundice.

Indications: jaundice due to damp heat, and acute jaundice-infectious hepatitis.

Notes: Experiments have shown that *yinchenhao* can (1) protect the liver, (2) reduce transaminase, (3) benefit the gallbladder and reduce jaundice, (4) promote liver bile production and bile excretion, (5) be used as a general antiviral herb, and (6) be used as an adjuvant herb to treat liver and gallbladder diseases.

Yinchenhao is particularly good at clearing damp heat in the liver and gallbladder, and is often used to treat damp-heat jaundice.

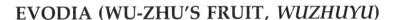

EVODIA (WU-ZHU'S FRUIT, *WUZHUYU*)

In ancient China, it was customary for a smaller and weaker kingdom to pay tribute to a larger and stronger kingdom in order to avoid war between the two kingdoms. Thus, Wu Kingdom, which was small and weak, paid tribute every year to Chu Kingdom, which was much larger and stronger.

In the spring of a good year, the ambassador of Wu Kingdom brought an herb as a New Year present to the king of Chu Kingdom, and told the king that it was called "Herb of Wu Kingdom" because it was the kingdom's national herb. But the king was visibly offended and declined the gift.

"How could a small and weak kingdom like Wu Kingdom have a national herb? I don't accept it as a present," said the king.

The ambassador was terribly humiliated and ready to return to his own country with the "Herb of Wu Kingdom," but a doctor in Chu Kingdom by the name of Dr. Zhu privately persuaded the ambassador to give the herb to him. Dr. Zhu planted the seeds, and one year later, the "Herb of Wu Kingdom" had become readily available in Chu Kingdom.

One day the king of Chu Kingdom suffered severe abdominal pain, so Dr. Zhu decocted the "Herb of Wu Kingdom" and gave the king the soup, which cured the king's abdominal pain instantly. The king was delighted. He then asked Dr. Zhu the name of the herb and was told that it was the "Herb of Wu Kingdom." Realizing the value of the herb, the king changed the name to "Wu-Zhu's Fruit." The king gave three reasons for the new name: First, the herb was a fruit; second, it was originally the herb of Wu Kingdom; and third, it was Dr. Zhu who had planted the herb in his kingdom.

Chinese: *Wuzhuyu* (Wu-Zhu's Fruit).
Re: 2280.

吴茱萸

Common name: evodia.
Family: Rutaceae.
Chinese name: evodia of Wu (so named because the herb grown in the Wu district is generally considered the best).

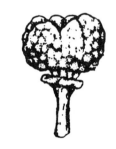

Scientific names: Euodia rutaecarpa (Juss.) Benth., Euodia rutaecarpa (Juss.) Benth. var. officinalis (Dode) Huang, and Euodia rutaecarpa (Juss.) Benth. var. bodinieri (Dode) Huang.
Pharmaceutical name: Fructus Euodiae.
Part used: unripe fruit.
Dosage: 5 g.
Flavor: pungent.
Energy: warm.

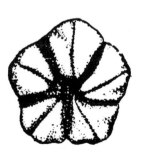

Class: 4, herbs to reduce cold sensations inside the body.
Meridians: liver, kidneys, spleen, and stomach.
Actions: to warm up the internal regions, disperse cold, relieve vomiting, and relieve pain.
Indications: cold abdominal pain, vomiting, diarrhea, and headache.

98

Notes: *Wuzhuyu* is particularly good for warming the liver and spleen and for relieving pain; it is frequently used to treat deficiency cold of the stomach and spleen and cold liver with hernial pain in the lower abdomen, as well as menstrual pain, and headache in the top of the head.

Huanglian (yellow-pearl rhizome) and *wuzhuyu* can be decocted together to treat pain in the ribs, excessive stomach acid, and belching, associated with "liver fire."

GREY ATRACTYLODES (GREY RHIZOME, *CANGZHU*)

Once a knowledgeable old nun boasted that she could cure all sorts of illnesses with herbs. But, being cunning and greedy in nature, this nun treated only rich patients, turning away any poor patients who could not afford the herbs. The nun did not pick the herbs herself, but instead ordered a younger nun to do the chore for her.

Then one day, a poor fellow who suffered from rheumatism in the legs, with both legs swollen and painful, came to see the nun, but she turned him away because he could not pay for the herbs. The young nun, being kind in nature but knowing little or nothing about herbs, then gave the fellow an herb she had picked without knowing what it was good for.

The fellow went home and decocted the herb, which by chance cured his legs. When he came back to thank the old nun, she was naturally taken aback. The old nun remembered that she had not given any herbs to this patient, so how could he be cured? She asked the patient for details, and discovered that it was the young nun who had given him the herb. She immediately expelled the young nun, who then went home and began to use that herb to treat patients with swollen and painful legs.

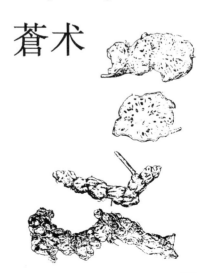

Chinese: *Cangzhu* (Grey Rhizome).
Re: 2174.
Common name: grey atractylode.
Family: Compositae.
Chinese name: grey essence (literal translation).
Scientific names: Atractylodes lancea (Thunb.) D.C. and Atractylodes chinensis (D.C.) Koidz.
Pharmaceutical name: Rhizoma Atractylodis.
Part used: rhizome.
Dosage: 10 g.
Flavor: pungent and bitter.
Energy: warm.

蒼术

Class: 5, herbs to remove dampness in the body.

Meridians: spleen and stomach.

Actions: to dry up dampness, expel wind, relieve pain, and sharpen vision.

Indications: rheumatism, weak legs, night blindness, and itchy skin.

Notes: Experiments have shown that *changzhu* can reduce blood sugar, and it contains volatile oils.

Cangzhu can be decocted with *huangbai* (yellow bark) to clear heat and dry dampness. This combination is considered good for pain in the lower region associated with damp heat, such as with weakened legs and eczema.

HARE'S EAR (WHO'S FIREWOOD, *CHAIHU*)

A governor by the name of Who had hired a young fellow as his domestic servant. This servant suffered from a disease with alternating fever and chills, and profuse perspiration. Since the young fellow was so ill and could not work, Governor Who dismissed him.

Having no place to go, this young servant wandered to a nearby pond. After lying by the pond for a few hours, the young servant began to feel thirsty and hungry, so he instinctively began to drink some dirty water from the pond and to eat some plants growing alongside it. The plants he ate were the ones that seemed the most edible under the circumstances.

The servant managed to survive by drinking water from the pond and eating these plants. Then strangely enough, on the seventh day, he began to regain strength and felt able to work again, so he went back to Governor Who. Surprised to see his former servant alive and well, Governor Who gave him his old job back.

One year later, Governor Who's only son suffered from a disease with alternating fever and chills, and profuse perspiration—the same disease his young servant had had the year before. Governor Who ordered his young servant to go to the pond to pick the plant that he had eaten when he was ill. The servant decocted the plant and the son's disease was cured within seven days. Governor Who named the herb "Who's firewood" after himself and because the plant was normally used as firewood.

Chinese: *Chaihu* (Who's Firewood).

Re: 3763.

柴胡

Common name: hare's ear.

Family: Umbelliferae.

Chinese name: wood and vegetable (so named because when the roots are

100

young and tender, they can be eaten as a vegetable, and when old, they are used as an herb).

Scientific names: Bupleurum chinense DC. and Bupleurum Scorzonerifolium Willd.

Pharmaceutical name: Radix Bupleuri.

Part used: root.

Dosage: 6 g.

Flavor: bitter.

Energy: slightly cold.

Class: 1, herbs to induce perspiration.

Meridians: liver, gallbladder, pericardium, and *sanjiao* (including the thoracic, abdominal, and pelvic cavities).

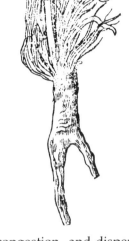

Actions: to elevate yang, disperse heat, relieve congestion, and disperse liver energy.

Indications: malaria, rib pain, irregular menstrual flow, and prolapse of the anus.

Notes: Experiments have shown that *chaihu* has six major actions: It can (1) reinforce the resistance of capillary vessels, (2) protect the liver, (3) benefit the gallbladder and reduce jaundice, (4) promote liver bile production and bile excretion, (5) treat fatty liver, and (6) soften and shrink the liver and the spleen.

Chaihu can elevate and disperse rather forcefully, which is why when used in large quantities, it may cause negative effects. *Chaihu* is basically a yang herb, and as such, it is very flexible, and can be combined with various herbs to produce different effects. For example, *chaihu* can be combined with *gegen* (radix puerariae) to induce perspiration and relax the superficial regions, with *changshan* (radix dichroae) to cure malaria, and with *huangqin* (radix scutellariae) to relax the superficial regions and sedate heat.

JAPANESE HONEYSUCKLE (GOLD-SILVER FLOWER, *JINYINHUA*)

There lived a young couple in a small village with two twin girls; one was named Golden Flower and the other Silver Flower. The twin girls, who had always loved each other, grew up to be very close, and had promised each other that they would never get married and would never separate from each other.

101

Not long after they had passed their seventeenth birthdays, Golden Flower suddenly fell ill, with a high fever and red spots all over her body.

"This is a contagious disease and there is no cure for it. Everybody should keep away from the patient," warned the doctor who made the diagnosis.

But Silver Flower insisted on staying close to her sister no matter what, and nobody could convince her otherwise.

However, the doctor was right; it was indeed a contagious disease, as the twin sisters died a few days later and were buried together.

In the spring of the following year, all kinds of plants were growing all over the graveyard, but nothing grew on the graves of the twin sisters, except for one plant with an abundance of yellow and white flowers. People in the village were very curious about this strange phenomenon, and some were even convinced that the twin sisters had turned into the flowers.

At the time when the plant was in full blossom, two little twin girls in the village fell ill with high fever and red spots all over their bodies—with exactly the same disease that killed Golden Flower and Silver Flower. The parents called on the same doctor to treat their little girls, and the doctor gave the same diagnosis.

Although they were told that there was no cure for the disease, the parents went ahead and picked the flowers that grew on the graves of the two deceased sisters and decocted them for their daughters to drink. The two little girls soon recovered from their illness to enjoy their happiness once again.

The people in the village named the herb after the deceased twin sisters, calling it "gold-silver flower."

Chinese: *Jinyinhua* (Gold-Silver Flower).
Re: 2894.
Common name: Japanese honeysuckle.
Family: Caprifoliaceae.
Chinese name: gold-silver flower (so named because it has both colors).
Scientific names: Lonicera japonica Thunb., Lonicera hypoglauca Miq., Lonicera confusa DC., and Lonicera dasystyle Rehd.
Pharmaceutical name: Flos Lonicerae.
Part used: buds.
Dosage: 12 g.
Flavor: sweet.
Energy: cold.

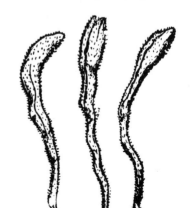

金銀花

102

Class: 2, herbs to reduce excessive heat inside the body.

Meridians: lungs, stomach, heart, and spleen.

Actions: to clear up heat, counteract toxic effects, cool down the blood, and disperse wind and heat.

Indications: carbuncles, dysentery, and sore throat with swelling.

Notes: Experiments have shown that *jinyinhua* can produce five major effects: It can (1) protect the liver, (2) inhibit influenza, (3) inhibit mumps, (4) reduce blood fat, and (5) be used as an antibacterial herb.

In addition, since this herb contains lonicerin, saponin, and inositol, and has been found to possess antibacterial and antiviral effects, it is now being widely used to treat the common cold, influenza, cystitis, arthritis, eye and throat infections, and contagious hepatitis.

KUDZU VINE (GE'S ROOT, *GEGEN*)

Mr. Ge was a high government official for many years, but when the government was overthrown by rebels, the members of the Ge family were all killed, except for Mr. Ge's oldest son, who had managed to escape.

An old herbalist was asleep when he heard someone screaming for help; he opened the window and saw a child about ten years old standing outside the door. The old herbalist opened the door to let him in.

"What is the matter?" asked the old herbalist.

The child explained what had happened to his family and said that he was the Ge's root, meaning that he was the only survivor in the family to carry the name of Ge to posterity.

The old herbalist was sympathetic and agreed to adopt him. The two would go to the mountain nearby to collect herbs every day, but there was one particular plant that they collected the most, whose root was especially good for neck pain and fever. Since this herb had no name, the people in the village called it "Ge's root" after the young boy and to commemorate the Ge family, who had served the government so faithfully.

Chinese: *Gegen* (Ge's Root). 葛根

Re: 4796.

Common name: root of lobed kudzu-vine.

Family: Leguminosae.

Chinese name: root of lobed kudzu-vine.

Scientific names: Pueraria lobata (Wild.) Ohwi and Pueraria thomsanii Benth.

Pharmaceutical name: Radix Puerariae.

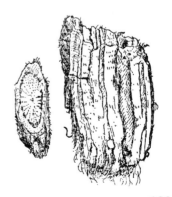

103

Part used: root.
Dosage: 10 to 25 g.
Flavor: sweet and pungent.
Energy: neutral.
Class: 1, herbs to induce perspiration.
Meridians: lungs and stomach.
Actions: to induce perspiration, clear heat, facilitate measles eruption, elevate clear energy, and relieve diarrhea.
Indications: measles prior to eruptions, diarrhea (better used in roasted form), headache in forehead, and stiff neck.
Notes: Experiments have shown that *gegen* can (1) expand coronary arteries and prevent angina pectoris, (2) reduce heat and bring down blood pressure, and (3) reduce blood sugar.

In addition, from a traditional point of view, *gegen* is good for relaxing muscles, reducing heat, facilitating measles eruptions, producing fluids, and quenching thirst. *Gegen* can be combined with *mahuang* to treat stiffness in the back of the neck.

LICORICE (SWEET ROOT, *GANCAO*)

A popular herbalist had left home to make house calls and in over a month had still not returned. This was naturally causing anxiety among his patients who had been coming to his home for treatment. His wife was very concerned about these patients and decided to do something about it.

Since she knew little to nothing about herbs, she began to taste them all—she tasted sour herbs, bitter herbs, salty herbs, pungent herbs, and sweet herbs. Thinking that most people would prefer sweet herbs, she decided to give all the patients the same sweet herb.

This sweet herb produced good results, and more and more patients came back to get more of it. In fact, the business became much better in the absence of the herbalist, which puzzled him a great deal upon his return.

Wondering how this sweet herb could bring about such good results, the herbalist decided to continue giving it to all the patients who came to see him. He found that the herb was most effective for low energy, cough, pain, and fatigue, and he called it "sweet herb" because it tasted sweet.

Chinese: *Gancao* (Sweet Root). 甘草
Re: 1187.
Common name: licorice.
Family: Leguminosae.

104

Chinese name: sweet grass (so named because it is a typical sweet herb).

Scientific names: Glycyrrhiza uralensis Fisch., Glycyrrhiza inflata Bat., and Glycyrrhiza Glabra L.

Pharmaceutical name: Radix Glycyrrhizae.

Parts used: root and tuberous root.

Dosage: 5 g.

Flavor: sweet.

Energy: neutral.

Class: 16, herbs to correct deficiencies.

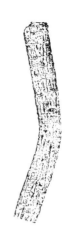

Meridians: twelve meridians.

Actions: to tone up the spleen, benefit energy, produce fluids, detoxicate, harmonize various herbs, and slow down the advancement of symptoms.

Indications: spleen and stomach weakness, dry cough, sore throat, acute abdominal pain, carbuncles, swelling, and poisoning.

Notes: Experiments have shown that *gancao* can produce five major effects: It can (1) protect the liver, (2) produce adrenocortical hormones, (3) inhibit influenza, (4) be effective for leukemia, and (5) reduce blood fat.

LILY-FLOWERED MAGNOLIA (BARBARIAN BUD, *XINYI*)

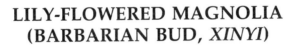

A government official suffered from a nose disease, which troubled him a great deal, because the nasal discharge smelled awful and constantly blocked his nose, forcing him to breathe through his mouth. He had sought help from many herbalists, but none seemed to be able to help him. His friends advised him to retire and tour the countryside to get fresh air, which they thought might give him more relief than any herbs could.

Since he was close to retirement anyway, he decided to follow his friends' advice. He took an early retirement and soon after embarked on a tour to the frontier. There, he met a frontiersman who was an herbalist, who gave him an herbal remedy for nasal disorders. After using it for a while, it cured his condition.

The government official brought the seeds of the herb back with him to grow in his own garden. When people asked him what the herb was, he told them that it was called "barbarian bud." Why? Because the Chinese have always called frontiersmen barbarians, and the bud of the plant is used as the herb.

Chinese: *Xinyi* (Barbarian Bud).
Re: 2354.
Common name: lily-flowered magnolia.
Family: Magnoliaceae.
Chinese name: pungent magnolia.
Scientific names: Magnolia biondii Pamp., Magnolia denudata Desr., and Magnolia liliflora Desr.
Pharmaceutical name: Flos Magnoliae.
Part used: dried buds.
Dosage: 3 to 10 g.
Flavor: pungent.
Energy: warm.
Class: 1, herbs to induce perspiration.
Meridians: lungs and stomach.

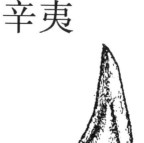
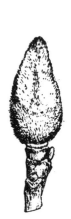

Actions: to expel wind, disperse cold, and open nasal passages.

Indications: thick nasal discharge, headache, and sinusitis.

Notes: *Xinyi* travels to the face and enters the nose in particular, which is why it is an effective herb for symptoms of the nose.

Xinyi can be combined with *huangqin* and *cangerzi* to treat heat-predominating symptoms of the nose.

MISTLETOE (MULBERRY PARASITE, *SANGJISHENG*)

The son of a wealthy man suffered from severe rheumatism. Since there was no cure, he had been bedridden for many years. The wealthy man heard about an herbalist living on a farm about five hundred miles away, so he sent his servant to buy some herbs from him.

Each time it would take the servant three weeks to get to the herbalist and back. The servant had made many trips and brought back over a hundred bags of herbs, but the wealthy man's son was still bedridden and showed not the slightest improvement.

One day when it was snowing very heavily, the servant was on his routine trip to the herbalist. He felt unusually exhausted along the way, so he stopped to rest under a white mulberry plant. He spotted a plant grow-

106

ing on the white mulberry that looked like the herb he brought home each time. Suddenly he thought, "Why don't I pick this plant and bring it home and tell the boss it's from the herbalist? Nothing has worked for his son's condition anyway." So the servant picked the plant and brought it home.

Since this had proven to be very convenient for the servant, he repeated it over the next two months. Strangely enough, after taking the plant picked by the servant, the wealthy man's son gradually recovered.

Seeing that the herb had cured his son, the wealthy man wanted to know its name. The servant told him that the herb was called "mulberry parasite," because it was a parasitic plant living on the white mulberry.

Chinese: _Sangjisheng_ (Mulberry Parasite). **Re:** 4046.

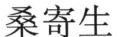

Common name: herb of colored mistletoe.

Family: Loranthaceae.

Chinese name: mulberry parasitic herb (so named because it is parasitic on mulberry plants).

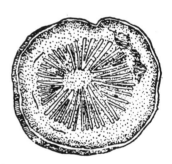

Scientific names: Loranthus parasiticus (L.) Merr., Viscum coloratum (Kom.) Nakai, and Loranthus gracilifolius Schult.

Pharmaceutical names: Ramulus Loranthi or Ramus Loranthi (Sangjisheng) and Herba Visci or Ramus Visci cum Folio (Hujisheng).

Part used: stalks.

Dosage: 10 g.

Flavor: bitter.

Energy: neutral.

Class: 16, herbs to correct deficiencies.

Meridians: liver and kidneys.

Actions: to nourish blood, expel wind, strengthen tendons and bones, secure fetus, and promote milk secretion.

Indications: blood deficiency, lumbago, weak legs, insecure fetus, and shortage of milk secretion.

Notes: Experiments have shown that _sangjisheng_ can produce seven major effects: It can (1) expand coronary arteries and prevent angina pectoris, (2) bring down blood pressure by tonification, (3) inhibit influenza, (4) reduce blood fat, (5) be generally effective in reducing blood pressure, (6) relieve pain, and (7) be used as an antirheumatic herb.

PSEUDOGINSENG (THREE-SEVEN ROOT, *SANQI*)

Two good friends promised one another that they would always help each other, like good brothers. In fact, people even started calling them brothers.

One day the younger brother suffered a severe nosebleed that wouldn't stop. So the older brother immediately rushed home to pick some herbs from his backyard and decocted them for the younger brother to drink, which stopped his nosebleed instantly. The younger brother later picked a branch to plant in his own backyard, just in case he should need it in the future.

One year later, the son of a government official suffered a severe nosebleed, so the younger brother immediately rushed to his garden to pick the herb to give it to the government official, promising that it would work. The government official decocted the herb and gave his son the soup, but it failed to stop his nosebleed. The government official was furious and the younger brother felt terribly humiliated. He went to confront his older brother, who explained that in order for the herb to be effective, the plant had to be between three and seven years old. Thus, the plant is called "three-seven root," as the root is used as the herb.

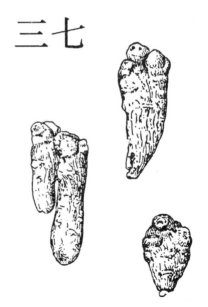

Chinese: *Sanqi* (Three-Seven Root).
Re: 0096.
Common name: pseudoginseng.
Family: Araliaceae.
Chinese name: three-seven and mountain paint (so named because this plant has three leaves on the left and four on the right, and it can heal boils like paint).
Scientific name: Panax notoginseng (Burk.) F. H. Chen.
Pharmaceutical name: Radix Notoginseng.
Part used: root.
Dosage: 8 g.
Flavor: sweet and slightly bitter.
Energy: warm.
Class: 12, herbs to regulate blood.
Meridians: liver and stomach.
Actions: to arrest bleeding of various kinds, promote blood circulation, heal swelling, and relieve pain.
Indications: bleeding of various kinds.
Notes: Experiments have shown that *sanqi* can produce four major effects:

108

It can (1) expand coronary arteries, (2) prevent angina pectoris, (3) increase and protect blood platelets, and (4) be an effective coagulant and arrest bleeding (as a hemostatic).

Sanqi can relieve pain and reduce swelling, and is often used to treat injuries. For best results, it should be applied in powder form.

RHUBARB (GREATER YELLOW ROOT, *DAHUANG*)

There was an herbalist who was called Mr. Five Yellow because he was known to have mastered five yellow herbs—yellow bark, yellow essence, greater yellow root, yellow root, and yellow pearl rhizome. This herbalist applied the five yellow herbs exclusively to treat diseases.

Mr. Five Yellow went to pick herbs every year in the country and often stayed in the house of Mr. Ma. The two had been friends for a couple of decades.

One spring when Mr. Five Yellow went to pick herbs, he found that Mr. Ma's house was gone and was told by a neighbor that it had burned down in a fire. His wife and children had died in the fire and Mr. Ma was living alone in a cave on the mountain.

Mr. Five Yellow climbed the mountain and found his friend and asked him whether he wanted to work with him. Mr. Ma agreed and from that time on, the two friends picked herbs together and lived together.

Mr. Five Yellow was an herbalist, but Mr. Ma was not; Mr. Ma wanted to become an herbalist and treat patients, but Mr. Five Yellow tried to persuade him not to.

"You are not careful enough to become an herbalist," Mr. Five Yellow told his friend, but Mr. Ma was not convinced.

One day while Mr. Five Yellow was away, Mr. Ma started treating patients on his own, and obtained good results initially. One day, however, a woman came to see him for diarrhea, who looked very weak and pale. Mr. Ma remembered that his friend often used yellow root to treat diarrhea, so he decocted greater yellow root for the patient to drink. But, after drinking the soup, the patient got much worse and almost died from severe diarrhea.

Mr. Ma did not know what had gone wrong. When his friend returned, Mr. Ma told Mr. Five Yellow what had happened. Mr. Five Yellow immediately knew that Mr. Ma had used the wrong herb, because there were two yellow roots, one for diarrhea and one for constipation. Yellow root was good for diarrhea, whereas greater yellow root was good for constipation.

109

Chinese: *Dahuang* (Greater Yellow Root). Re: 0188.

大黃

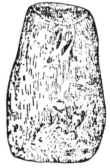

Common name: rhubarb.

Family: Polygonaceae.

Chinese name: greater yellowness (so named because it is yellow and produces a greater effect than other yellow herbs); also called "a general."

Scientific names: Rheum palmatum L., Rheum tanguticum Maxim. ex Balf., and Rheum officinale Baill.

Pharmaceutical name: Radix Et Rhizoma Rhei.

Parts used: root and rhizome.

Dosage: 10 g.

Flavor: bitter.

Energy: cold.

Class: 8, herbs to induce bowel movements.

Meridians: spleen, stomach, pericardium, liver, and large intestine.

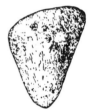

Actions: to attack accumulations, sedate fire, counteract toxic effects, and remove coagulations.

Indications: excess heat in the stomach and intestine, nosebleed, coagulation, vomiting of blood, and suppression of menstruation.

Notes: Experiments have indicated that *dahuang* can produce seven major effects: It can (1) be used as an effective digestive, (2) be effective for promoting gastrointestinal peristalsis, (3) promote bowel movements, (4) benefit the gallbladder and reduce jaundice, (5) increase and protect blood platelets, (6) inhibit influenza, and (7) treat bacteria.

In addition, *dahuang* contains anthraquinone glycosides, which accounts for its being used as a laxative; but it also contains tannin that obstructs bowel movements, which explains why, when taken in small doses, it can cause constipation.

Modern research has also revealed that *dahuang* contains bacterides, which is why this herb has often been used to treat acute contagious hepatitis with jaundice and constipation, dysentery, and suppression of menstruation due to blood coagulations.

Aside from being a strong and forceful herb in inducing bowel movements, this herb can also activate the blood, remove blood coagulations, promote meridian energy flow, and detoxicate, and it is good for vomiting blood, nosebleed, suppression of menstruation, and swelling.

Dahuang and *huangqin* (skullcap) can be decocted together to improve the

110

effect of sedating heat. *Dahuang* and *fanxieye* (folium sennae) are both cold laxatives. But *dahuang* produces a more drastic action, whereas the power of *fanxieye* varies with the quantities consumed and the methods used in taking it. Making tea out of *fanxieye* will produce more drastic actions than by decocting it.

SEALWORT (YELLOW ESSENCE, *HUANGJING*)

Sometime in the third century A.D., when Dr. Hua Duo was picking herbs on a mountain, he saw two strong young men chasing after a young girl; the girl was about seventeen years old, but the two strong young men could not catch her, because they couldn't run as fast as she could. This greatly puzzled Dr. Hua Duo, who inquired about the young girl. The two young men told Dr. Hua Duo that the girl had escaped from a foster home three years before and no one had known of her whereabouts until now.

Wanting to know more about this girl, particularly about what she had been eating that had made her so energetic, Dr. Hua Duo devised a scheme to catch her. He prepared a bowl of food and placed it in a cave; then he hid in a bush to wait for the girl to come. A few hours later, the girl came to eat the food, and Dr. Hua Duo immediately blocked the cave to keep her from escaping. When he questioned her, the young girl told him that she had been eating the big fleshy roots of a plant, which looked very much like a chicken.

After letting the girl go, Dr. Hua Duo found the plant and dug out the fleshy roots. He later named the plant "the yellow essence," because it was yellow and as pure as essence.

Chinese: *Huangjing* (Yellow Essence). 黄精

Re: 4157.

Common name: sealwort.

Family: Liliaceae.

Chinese name: yellow pure substance.

Scientific names: Polygonatum kingianum Coll. et Hemsl., Polygonatum sibiricum Red, and Polygonatum cyrtonema Hua.

Pharmaceutical name: Rhizoma Polygonati.

Part used: underground rhizome.

Dosage: 10 to 20 g.

Flavor: sweet.

Energy: neutral.

Class: 16, herbs to correct deficiencies.

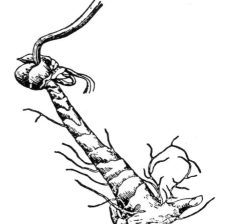

111

Meridians: spleen, lungs, and stomach.

Actions: to water (to increase yin energy) and lubricate the heart and lungs, tone up the middle region, benefit energy, and fill in semen and marrow.

Indications: yin deficiency, blood deficiency, grey hair, dry throat, thirst, and diabetes.

Notes: Experiments have indicated that *huangjing* can produce five major effects: It can (1) bring down blood pressure by tonification, (2) protect the liver, (3) treat fatty liver, (4) reduce blood sugar, and (5) reduce blood fat.

Huangjing is an important spleen tonic. It can also lubricate the lungs, and is therefore good for cough due to dry lungs, lung deficiencies, diabetes, and deficiency after illness.

Huangjing is sticky and for this reason, it should be decocted for a longer period of time than most other herbs in order to extract its active ingredients.

SELF-HEAL (SEE-ME-NOT-AFTER-SUMMER, *XIAKUCAO*)

The mother of a mayor suffered from scrofula with a swollen neck. All the doctors said there was no cure for it. One day, however, an herbalist came along who told the mayor that he knew of an herb that could cure the disease.

The herbalist climbed a nearby mountain to pick the herb and brought it to the mayor for decoction, and it indeed cured the patient.

Prior to his departure, the herbalist told the mayor that the herb grew only during the summer, and that it would be gone when the summer was over.

In the winter of the following year, the governor suffered from scrofula with a swollen neck. The mayor was eager to help, so he told the governor about the herb that had cured his mother. The mayor then climbed the mountain to pick the plants, but he couldn't find any growing there and returned home empty-handed. Naturally, the governor was terribly disappointed and the mayor felt very embarrassed.

When the herbalist returned in the summer, the mayor blamed him for his failure to find the herb.

"I made it a point to tell you before I left that this herb cannot be found after the summer is over," said the herbalist. And so, the herb was named "see-me-not-after-summer" to remind herbalists that it grows only during the summer.

Chinese: *Xiakucao* (See-Me-Not-After-Summer). 夏枯草
Re: 3752.
Common name: fruit spike of common self-heal.
Family: Labiatae.

112

Chinese name: summer withering grass.
Scientific name: Prunella vulgaris L.
Pharmaceutical name: Spica Prunellae.
Part used: ear of fruit (fruit spike).
Dosage: 10 to 30 g.
Flavor: slightly bitter.
Energy: cool.
Class: 2, herbs to reduce excessive heat inside the body.
Meridians: liver and gallbladder.
Actions: to calm down the liver, clear up heat, soften up hardness, and disperse congestion.
Indications: headache, pinkeye, carbuncles of the head, and scrofula.
Notes: Experiments have shown that this herb can produce four major effects: It can (1) clear heat and bring down blood pressure, (2) soften and shrink the liver and the spleen, (3) treat various types of cancers, and (4) treat tuberculosis.

SIBERIAN MOTHERWORT
(GOOD-FOR-MOTHER, *YIMUCAO*)

A mother was living with her ten-year-old son. The mother had been ill since her child was born, with abdominal pain and irregular menstruation due to blood coagulation after childbirth. Seeing that his mother had been suffering for so long, the child tried to persuade her to see a doctor. But the mother always declined, saying that they couldn't afford it.

So the child went to see an herbalist on his own. He bought an herb from him, and decocted it for his mother. After taking it, she felt a little better. The child then went back to the herbalist and asked him if he could cure his mother. The herbalist said yes but it would cost him five hundred pounds of rice. This saddened the child, as he knew that there was no way that he could come up with that much rice. Then suddenly the child had an idea, and he told the herbalist that he would pay him the five hundred pounds of rice *after* his mother had been cured. The herbalist agreed to the child's proposal.

At midnight, the herbalist climbed the mountain to dig up the herb, with the child secretly following behind him. After the herbalist had gone home with the plants, the child stayed on to dig up some more and then brought them home to his mother.

The next day, the herbalist brought the herb to the child's house, but the child told him that he hadn't been able to come up with the five hundred pounds of rice. So the herbalist left, taking the herb with him.

113

The child's mother was cured by the herb her child had picked, and the herb has been called "good-for-mother" ever since.

Chinese: *Yimucao* (Good-for-Mother).
Re: 4016.
Common name: Siberian motherwort.
Family: Labiatae.
Chinese name: mother's herb (so named because this herb can benefit mothers in many ways, but in menstrual disorders in particular).
Scientific name: Leonurus heterophyllus Sweet.
Pharmaceutical name: Herba Leonuri.
Part used: whole plant.
Dosage: 10 g.
Flavor: bitter and pungent.
Energy: neutral.
Class: 12, herbs to regulate blood.
Meridians: pericardium and liver.

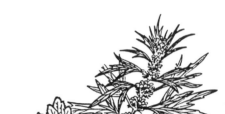

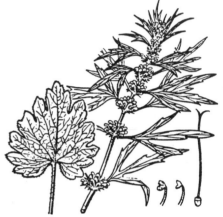

Actions: to activate the blood, regulate menstruation, disperse coagulations, and heal edema.
Indications: abdominal pain due to blood coagulations after childbirth, irregular menstruation, and vaginal bleeding.
Notes: Experiments have shown that *yimucao* can activate the blood and bring down blood pressure, regulate menstruation, and induce contraction of the uterus and labor. *Yimucao* contains benzoic acid.

TEASEL (FRACTURE HEALER, *XUDUAN*)

Once an herbalist was passing through a small village when he heard someone crying; he stopped to inquire about the details and was told that the child lying on the floor was dead and that the crying woman was his mother.

The herbalist took the pulse of the child and told the mother that he was still alive. He took out a bottle of herbal tablets from his briefcase, and put ten tiny tablets in the child's mouth; he then washed them down with a

114

cup of warm water. Hours later, the child regained consciousness. The herbalist told the mother that her child should fully recover within a month.

There was an herb shop in the village operated by a powerful and wealthy man who had always monopolized the herb business in the village. When this man heard about the incident, he tried to convince the herbalist to give him the tablets, but the herbalist always declined. So finally he sent two big strong fellows over to beat up the herbalist and break his legs.

Although the herbalist was hurt and had two broken legs, he still had the strength to climb the mountain to pick an herb that would heal his broken legs. A couple of months later, when the herbalist's legs had completely healed, he was able to resume treating patients.

Seeing that the herbalist could walk again and thinking that his legs had not actually been broken, the owner of the herb shop was furious. This time when he instructed the two big fellows to beat up the herbalist, he wanted them to make sure that his legs were really broken. So they beat him up once more and the herbalist became crippled again.

The herbalist could not climb the mountain to pick the herb this time; so, instead, he instructed a young man to do it for him. The young man did and once again the herbalist recovered a couple of months later.

When the owner of the herb shop learned that the herbalist had recovered from his broken legs, he instructed the two big fellows to kill him.

After the herbalist's death, the young man taught the people in the village how to heal broken bones by using the herb that the herbalist had used to heal himself; this young man named the herb "fracture healer."

Chinese: _Xuduan_ (Fracture Healer).
Re: 4706.
Common name: teazel.
Family: Dipsacaceae.
Chinese name: reconnect broken parts.
Scientific name: Dipsacus asper Wall.
Pharmaceutical name: Radix Dipsaci.
Part used: root.
Dosage: 5 to 10 g.
Flavor: bitter and pungent.
Energy: slightly warm.
Classes: herbs to counteract rheumatism (class 3) and herbs to correct deficiencies (class 16).
Meridians: liver and kidneys.

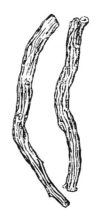

Actions: to tone up the liver and kidneys, strengthen loins and knees, connect tendons and bones, and secure fetus.

115

Indications: lumbago, soft legs, disconnected tendons and fracture, insecure fetus, and vaginal bleeding.

Notes: *Xuduan* can tonify the liver and kidneys, and strengthen tendons and bones to treat lumbago. It is a particularly effective herb for promoting energy and blood circulation and for treating fractures and vaginal bleeding.

CHINESE MAGNOLIAVINE FRUITS (FIVE-FLAVORED FRUIT, *WUWEIZI*)

Once a fellow suffered from tuberculosis and kept losing weight until he looked like a bamboo stick. The people in the small village where he lived wanted to get rid of him, because they thought that tuberculosis was highly contagious. One neighbor had suggested that they put him on a boat to die in the high seas, and another had hinted that he should be burned to death or killed with a knife.

Upon hearing of the plots against their son, the parents of the patient became very worried and then finally came up with an idea.

"Son, your dad and I love you very much, but we cannot help you in any other way except to take you to the mountain where you can hide from the people in the village. If you are lucky and recover from this illness, you can return home; but if you die, we will bury you as soon as we know about it," said his mother with tears in her eyes.

And so, this fellow was taken to the mountain and put in a cave to live on his own. He had managed to survive on the dried foods he had brought with him, but when they were all used up, he didn't have the strength to look for any more food. One day he had become so weak that he was ready to give up the struggle, and he started crying out loud.

Hearing his sobs, a hunter appeared at the entrance to the cave and asked him what was the matter. After the sick fellow explained his predicament, the hunter said, "I am just a hunter, not a doctor, so I am afraid I cannot help you. But I can pick some fruit for you to eat."

The fruit the hunter gave him lasted for ten days. At that point, the fellow had gradually regained enough strength to start picking the same fruit by himself.

In a few months, he had recovered from the tuberculosis and went home. When his parents saw him alive and well, at first they couldn't believe their eyes. Later when they asked him how he had managed to recover, he told them about the fruit. The whole village was in shock, and this fellow lived to be over one hundred years old.

116

Chinese: *Wuweizi* (Five-Flavor Seed). **Re:** 0772.

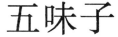

Common name: Chinese magnolia-vine fruits.

Family: Magnoliaceae.

Chinese name: five-flavored seed (so named because its bark and flesh are mixtures of sweet, sour, and salty flavors, and its kernel tastes pungent, bitter, and salty; hence, five flavors in one herb).

Scientific names: Schisandra chinensis (Turcz.) Baill. and Schisandra sphenanthera Rehd. et Wils.

Pharmaceutical name: Fructus Schisandrae.

Part used: ripe fruit.

Dosage: 5 g.

Flavor: all five, but predominantly sour.

Energy: warm.

Class: 17, herbs to constrict and obstruct movements.

Meridians: lungs and kidneys.

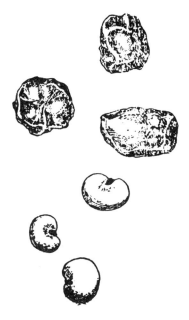

Actions: to water (increase yin energy in) kidneys, constrict lungs, produce fluids, check perspiration and diarrhea, and constrict semen.

Indications: asthma and cough, excessive perspiration, night sweats, diarrhea, seminal emission, and vaginal bleeding.

Notes: All herbs and foods have flavors; for example, grapes taste sour and sweet, ginseng tastes sweet and bitter, and green onions taste pungent. But very few foods or herbs have all of the five flavors—namely, sweet, sour, bitter, pungent, and salty—all at the same time. *Wuweizi* is one of these exceptions.

Experiments have shown that *wuweizi* can produce seven major effects: (1) It is effective for suppression of cough, (2) it is an effective heart tonic, (3) it is effective as a digestive, (4) it can increase acid, (5) it can reduce transaminase, (6) it can produce excitation, and (7) it can be used as an adjuvant herb to treat liver and gallbladder diseases.

Wuweizi can check excessive perspiration and constrict the lungs simultaneously, which is why it is often used to treat cough and asthma due to lung deficiency. In addition, this herb is often used to produce fluids and quench thirst, and in recent years it has also been used to treat insomnia, forgetfulness, and hepatitis.

117

LUCID GANODERMA (SPIRITUAL VEGETABLE MEAT, *LINGZHI*)

In a small village a long time ago there lived a dedicated student with a great ambition to pass the empirial examinations to become a government official. This student was so ambitious that the people in the village called him Mr. Ambition.

But having failed the empirial examinations a dozen times, Mr. Ambition decided to shift his ambition and become a Taoist monk instead. Enjoying longevity as a monk, he thought, was more important than becoming a government official. And so, Mr. Ambition put the mundane world behind him and went to stay in a temple on the mountain. There, he became a dedicated Taoist monk, fasting regularly and eating nothing but vegetables.

After having been a Taoist monk for less than a year, one day Mr. Ambition looked at himself in the mirror, and to his great astonishment, saw that he had lost so much weight that he looked as skinny as a stick. Mr. Ambition was so scared about his poor health that he immediately left the temple and returned to the mundane world.

Mr. Ambition had made a fortune not long after returning to the city through his construction company, but his fortune did not help him regain his good health. One day while building a large apartment building, Mr. Ambition's workers dug out a strange object from the ground. With its thick flesh and soft body, it almost looked like a huge human hand. Everyone was scared, but particularly Mr. Ambition. "Could this be a bad omen for me? Would the building collapse after its completion?" he worried. It was decided that a fortune-teller should be summoned to shed light on the situation.

"This object signals a real disaster for you, Mr. Ambition," said the fortune-teller.

"How can I prevent this disaster?" asked Mr. Ambition, with his face turning pale. "I would do anything."

After a long pause, the fortune-teller said, "Well, you could turn the upcoming disaster into good luck if you had the courage to eat that strange object."

Mr. Ambition was initially shocked at the suggestion, but later agreed to it, and ate the big fleshy object that night at dinner. It didn't taste as bad as he had anticipated it would; in fact, he somewhat enjoyed its taste.

A few days later, Mr. Ambition began to feel dramatic changes taking place in his body: His complexion had improved considerably, he had put on weight, his grey hair had returned to its original color, and he looked much younger than his age. And he really felt great!

Later that week, a Taoist monk passed by the construction site where Mr. Ambition was working. Spotting Mr. Ambition, he stopped and said to him, "Sir, you look different from other people. Did anything extraordinary happen to you recently? Have you eaten anything unusual? Let me take your pulse." Mr. Ambition sat down with the Taoist monk. After taking his pulse, the monk said, "Sir, did you possibly eat something that looks like a big human hand?" Mr. Ambition admitted that he had and told the monk the whole story. The monk said, "Sir, the strange object that you ate is an herb called 'spiritual vegetable meat,' and now that you've eaten it, you no longer belong to this mundane world. You ought to come with me to the temple on the mountain, where you can be a Taoist monk and enjoy immortality on earth."

Mr. Ambition took his advice and went with him to the temple, where he stayed for good.

Chinese: *Lingzhicao* (Spiritual Vegetable Meat).
Re: 2395.
Common name: lucid ganoderma and glossy ganoderma.
Family: Polyporaceae.
Chinese name: *lingzhi* (spiritual mushroom).
Scientific names: Ganoderma lucidum (Leyss. ex Fr.) Karst. and Ganoderma japonicum (Fr.) Lloyd.
Pharmaceutical name: Ganoderma Lucidum Seu Japonicum.
Part used: whole plant.
Dosage: 2 to 4 g in powder.
Flavor: sweet.
Energy: neutral.
Class: unclassified.
Meridians: undetermined.

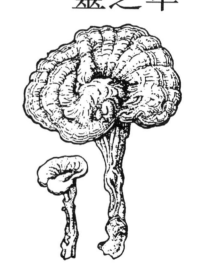

靈芝草

Actions: to benefit joints, protect the spirits, benefit pure energy, strengthen tendons and bones, and improve complexion.
Indications: deficiency fatigue, cough, asthma, insomnia, indigestion, deafness, chronic tracheitis, bronchial asthma, leukocytopenia, coronary heart disease, and irregular heartbeats.

Notes: Experiments indicate that *lingzhicao* can produce nine effects: It (1) is effective for asthma, (2) is an effective heart tonic, (3) can protect the liver, (4) can reduce transaminase, (5) can increase white blood cells, (6) can increase and protect blood platelets, (7) can sedate and inhibit, (8) can relieve pain, and (9) can reduce blood fat.

THREE APHRODISIAC HERBS

Fruit of Common Cnidium (Snake-Bed Seed, *Schechuangzi*), Chinese Cynomorium (Yang Locker, *Suoyang*), and Herb of Epimedium (Sexual Plant for Goats, *Yinyanghuo*)

A strange skin disease had attacked many people in a small village. The people with this disease felt itchy all over and had eruptions here and there, as well as rapidly spreading boils. The disease was regarded as highly contagious.

The people in the village knew that there was an herb growing on a small island about ten miles away that could cure the disease. But they also knew that poisonous snakes were in the habit of sleeping on this herb and there were many poisonous snakes on the island. So, naturally, most herbalists were too frightened to set foot on the island.

There was one brave young man who did decide to go. He prepared himself a big bag of rice and rowed a boat to the island. This young man never returned. A few months later, another brave young man did the same thing, and he, too, failed to return.

The people in the village had almost given up hope when a third brave young man said that he would go. But instead of going straight to the island, this young man went to a seaside temple, where he had heard there was a nun who was an expert at controlling snakes. The nun told the young man that poisonous snakes are afraid of realgar wine; she then gave him a bottle and he headed for the island.

Upon landing, the young man found the island to be full of poisonous snakes. He poured the realgar wine over the ground as he walked along, and the snakes all remained very still. When he came to the herb he was looking for, the young man had to push them aside, as several snakes were lying on the herb.

The young man finally returned to the village with the herb, which subsequently cured the people's strange skin disease. He named the herb "snake-bed seed" because the seeds of the plant are used as the herb and snakes sleep on the plant.

Chinese: *Shechuangzi* (Snake-Bed Seed).
Re: 4345.
Common name: fruit of common cnidium.

蛇床子

120

Family: Umbelliferae.
Chinese name: snake-bed seed.
Scientific name: Cnidium monnieri (L.) Cuss.
Pharmaceutical name: Fructus Cnidii.
Parts used: seeds and ripe fruit.
Dosage: 3 to 10 g.
Flavor: pungent and bitter.
Energy: warm.
Classes: herbs to correct deficiencies (class 16) and herbs for external applications (class 20).
Meridians: kidneys and *sanjiao.*

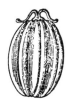

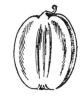

Actions: to destroy worms, dry up dampness, and strengthen yang.

Indications: chronic tinea and scabies, eczema involving scrotum, itchy genitals in women, and impotence.

Notes: Modern experiments indicate that *shechuangzi* can produce sex hormones. From the traditional point of view, this herb has been found to be slightly toxic.

*   *   *

Another herb that is good for improving sexual functions is *suoyang*. The Chinese name for this herb means "to lock the yang," with "yang" referring to a man's penis, and "to lock" meaning to control. Thus, the herb is used to control the actions of the penis.

Yinyanghuo is also good for improving sexual functions. The Chinese name for this herb means "sexual plant for goats," which originated from the following story. Once there was a shepherd who wondered why his goats were so sexually active. He started watching what they were eating and noticed that they consumed a great deal of one plant in particular, which he later named "sexual plant for goats."

All three aphrodisiac herbs can warm the kidneys and strengthen the yang to treat impotence, seminal emission, and premature ejaculation due to kidney yang deficiency. In terms of their differences (first) *suoyang* is a better herb to strengthen yang and promote bowel movements, which are essential in the treatment of constipation due to yang deficiency; (second) *shechuangzi* is a better herb for drying dampness and destroying worms, which is why it can be used to treat itch in the genital areas due to dampness, and also scabies and sores, chronic tinea, etc.; and (third) *yinyanghuo* can produce sexual hormones more quickly, and is also an effective herb for lumbago and arthritis and rheumatism in the legs.

121

Chinese: *Suoyang* (Yang Locker).
Re: 4976.
Common name: Chinese cynomorium.
Family: Cynomoriaceae.
Chinese name: yang locker.
Scientific name: Cynomorium songaricum Rupr.
Pharmaceutical names: Herba Cynomorii and Caulis Cynomorii.
Part used: fleshy stems.
Dosage: 2 to 4 g.
Flavor: sweet.
Energy: warm.
Class: 16, herbs to correct deficiencies.
Meridians: kidneys.

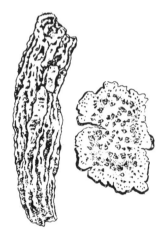

锁阳

Actions: to tone up kidneys, strengthen yang, benefit semen, and lubricate intestine.

Indications: impotence, constipation due to blood deficiency, and weak loins and knees.

Notes: *Suoyang* can tonify and assist yang to treat impotence, seminal emission, premature ejaculation, and weak loins and knees due to kidney yang deficiency on the one hand. On the other hand, it can also lubricate dryness and make the intestines smooth, which are essential in the treatment of deficiency constipation.

Chinese: *Yinyanghuo* (Sexual Plant for Goats).
Re: 4672.
Common name: herb of epimedium.
Family: Berberidaceae.
Chinese name: grass for goat's sexual drive.
Scientific names: Epimedium brevicornum Maxim., Epimedium koreanum Nakai, and Epimedium sagittatum (Sieb. et Zucc.) Maxim.
Pharmaceutical name: Herba Epimedii.
Part used: stalk leaves or whole plant.
Dosage: 4 to 15 g.
Flavor: pungent.
Energy: warm.

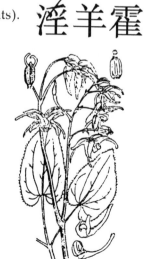

淫羊霍

122

Class: 16, herbs to correct deficiencies.

Meridians: liver and kidneys.

Actions: to tone up life door and strengthen tendons and bones. (Life door refers to yang energy in the kidneys that is responsible for male sexual capability.)

Indications: impotence, rheumatism, and hypertension.

Notes: Experiments indicate that *yinyanghuo* can bring down blood pressure by tonification, and can also produce sex hormones. When used to improve sexual functions in men, the leaves have stronger effects than the stalks. When used to treat hypertension, this herb can be decocted with *huangbai* (yellow bark), which is particularly effective for hypertension during menopause in women. *Yinyanghuo* is regarded as an effective herb to treat cold and damp rheumatism and hypertension due to kidney yang deficiency.

CHINESE HERBS NAMED AFTER THEIR COLORS

This category includes red, white, and green herbs, as well as one black herb.

Chinese: *Honghua.* 紅花

Re: 1999.

Common name: safflower.

Family: Compositae.

Chinese name: red flower (so named because of its color).

Scientific name: Carthamus tinctorius L.

Pharmaceutical name: Flos Carthami.

Part used: corolla.

Dosage: 6 g.

Flavor: pungent.

Energy: warm.

Class: 12, herbs to regulate blood.

Meridians: heart and liver.

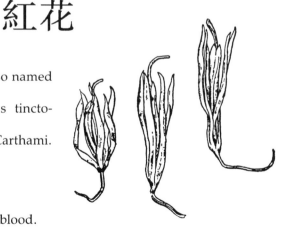

Actions: to activate blood, facilitate menstrual flow, disperse blood coagulations, and relieve pain.

Indications: menstrual pain, suppression of menstruation, dead fetus, swelling, and lochiostasis.

Notes: Experiments have shown that this herb can expand coronary arteries and prevent angina pectoris, activate the blood and bring down blood pressure, treat various types of cancers, and regulate menstruation.

123

Chinese: *Chishaoyao.* 赤芍

Re: 2225.

Common name: red peony root.

Family: Ranunculaceae.

Chinese name: red peony (so named due to its color).

Scientific name: Paeonia lactiflora Pall.

Pharmaceutical name: Radix Paeoniae Rubra.

Part used: root.

Dosage: 5 to 10 g.

Flavor: sour and bitter.

Energy: cool.

Class: 2, herbs to reduce excessive heat inside the body.

Meridians: liver and spleen.

Actions: to remove blood coagulations, relieve pain, cool the blood, and reduce swelling.

Indications: suppression of menses due to blood coagulation, abdominal obstructions in women, abdominal pain, pain in the ribs, nosebleeds, dysentery with blood in stools, pinkeye, and carbuncles.

Notes: Experiments indicate that *chishaoyao* is effective in inhibiting gastrointestinal peristalsis, and can also inhibit influenza. This herb should be avoided by those with blood deficiency.

Chishaoyao is often used to clear heat, cool the blood, activate the blood, remove coagulations, reduce swelling, relieve pain, and treat sores and ulcers.

Chinese: *Baizhi.* 白芷

Re: 1380.

Common name: angelica.

Family: Umbelliferae.

Chinese name: white rootlet (so named because the herb is white and shaped like a rootlet).

Scientific names: Angelica dahurica (Fisch. ex Hoffm.) Benth. et Hook. f., Angelica dahurica (Fisch. ex Hoffm.) Benth. et Hook. f. var., and taiwaniana (Boiss.) Shan et Yuan.

Pharmaceutical name: Radix Angelicae Dahuricae.

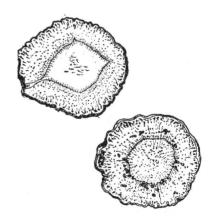

124

Part used: root.

Dosage: 5 g.

Flavor: pungent.

Energy: warm.

Classes: herbs to counteract rheumatism (class 3) and herbs to induce perspiration (class 1).

Meridians: lungs, stomach, and large intestine.

Actions: to induce perspiration, expel wind, heal swelling, and relieve pain.

Indications: headache, toothache, pain in the bony ridge of the eye socket, sinusitis, discharge of blood from the anus, and itch.

Notes: Experiments indicate that *baizhi* can produce excitation, and is also an effective herb for relief of pain. In addition, *baizhi* contains volatile oils, protein, carbohydrates, and fat, which make it readily eaten by insects.

Baizhi is a strong herb for relieving pain. It can also open cavities and drain off pus, and is often used to treat rhinitis, sinusitis, carbuncles, and burns.

Chinese: *Baiji.* 白及

Re: 1374.

Common name: amethyst orchid.

Family: Orchidaceae.

Chinese name: white orchid (so named due to its color).

Scientific name: Bletilla striata (Thunb.) Reichb.f.

Pharmaceutical name: Rhizoma (Tuber) Bletillae.

Part used: underground tuberous root.

Dosage: 10 to 20 g.

Flavor: bitter.

Energy: neutral.

Class: 12, herbs to regulate blood.

Meridians: lungs.

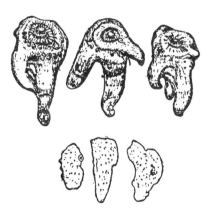

Actions: to arrest bleeding, constrict lungs, produce muscles, and heal wounds.

Indications: vomiting of blood, coughing up blood, nosebleeds, ulcers, and pulmonary tuberculosis.

Notes: Experiments indicate that *baiji* can produce four effects: (1) It can increase and protect blood platelets, (2) it is an effective coagulant, (3) it is an antituberculotic herb, and (4) it can arrest bleeding (as a hemostatic).

125

Chinese: *Baiwei.*
白薇

Re: 1394.

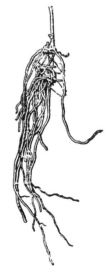

Common name: white rose.

Family: Asclepiadaceae.

Chinese name: white rose (so named due to its color).

Scientific names: Cynanchum atratum Bge. and Cynanchum versicolor Bge.

Pharmaceutical name: Radix Cynanchi Atrati.

Part used: root.

Dosage: 6 to 12 g.

Flavor: bitter and salty.

Energy: cold.

Class: 2, herbs to reduce excessive heat inside the body.

Meridians: undetermined.

Actions: to benefit yin, clear up heat, and cool blood.

Indications: periodic fever due to yin deficiency, and fever in warm-hot diseases.

Notes: *Baiwei* contains cynanchol.

Chinese: *Baizhu*
白术

Re: 1376.

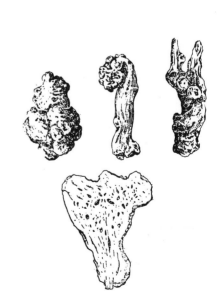

Common name: white atractylode.

Family: Compositae.

Chinese name: white atractylode (so named due to its color).

Scientific name: Atractylodes macrocephala Koidz.

Pharmaceutical name: Rhizoma Atractylodis.

Part used: rhizome.

Dosage: 5 g.

Flavor: sweet and bitter.

Energy: warm.

Class: 16, herbs to correct deficiencies.

Meridians: spleen and stomach.

126

Actions: to tone up energy, strengthen spleen, dry up dampness, benefit water, and check perspiration.

Indications: spleen deficiency, poor appetite, edema, and excessive perspiration.

Notes: Experiments indicate that *baizhu* can protect the liver, promote urination, and reduce blood sugar.

Chinese: *Qingpi* 青皮

Re: 2485.

Common name: green orange-peel.

Family: Rutaceae.

Chinese name: green peel (so named because of its color).

Scientific names: Citrus reticulata Blanco, Citrus tangerina Hortorum et Tanaka, Citrus unshiu Marcovitch, Citrus sinensis (L.) Osbeck-wilsonii Tanaka.

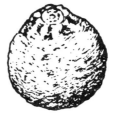
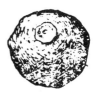

Pharmaceutical names: Pericarpium Citri Reticulate. Viride and Fructus Aurantii Immaturus.

Parts used: peel of unripe fruit, and fruit.

Dosage: 5 g.

Flavor: bitter and pungent.

Energy: warm.

Class: 11, herbs to regulate energy.

Meridians: liver and gallbladder.

Actions: to disperse energy congestion, disperse accumulations, promote energy flow, and relieve pain.

Indications: chest swelling and pain, and hernial pain in the lower abdomen.

Notes: This herb consists of the peel of unripe oranges. It is an effective herb for promoting energy circulation to relieve energy congestion in the liver and gallbladder, to relax the liver for the relief of pain, to break up energy, and to disperse congestion. It is a strong herb in promoting energy circulation, and is often used to treat pain in the chest and ribs, food stagnation, and energy congestion.

Chinese: *Qinghao.* 青蒿

Re: 2491.

Common name: southern wood.

Family: Compositae.

Chinese name: green evergreen artemisia (so named because the leaves and stems of this herb remain green in autumn, and it's similar to evergreen artemisia in shape).

Scientific names: Artemisia annua L. and Artemisia apiacea Hance.

Pharmaceutical name: Herba Artemisiae Chinghao.

Part used: rhizome.

Dosage: 6 g.

Flavor: bitter.

Energy: cold.

Class: 2, herbs to reduce excessive heat inside the body.

Meridians: liver and kidneys.

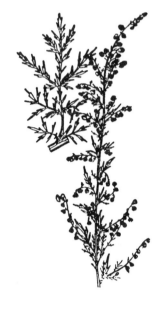

Actions: to relieve summer heat, clear up heat, and relieve hot sensations as if coming from the bones.

Indications: malaria, hot sensations, and scabies.

Notes: Experiments indicate that this herb can inhibit influenza. It is an aromatic herb. It is good for warm diseases in their later stages, hot sensations at night, and cold sensations in the morning.

Chinese: *Xuanshen.* 玄参

Re: 1542.

Common name: figwort.

Family: Scrophulariaceae.

Chinese name: dark ginseng (so named because its stalk looks like ginseng, but it's dark).

Scientific name: Scrophularia ningpoensis Hemsl.

Pharmaceutical name: Radix Scrophulariae.

Part used: tuberous root.

Dosage: 10 g.

Flavor: bitter and salty.

Energy: cold.

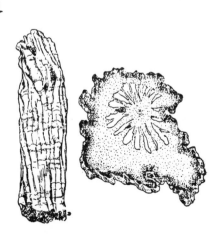

128

Classes: herbs to reduce excessive heat inside the body (class 2) and herbs for lubricating dry symptoms (class 6).

Meridians: lungs and kidneys.

Actions: to clear up heat, water yin (increase yin energy), bring down fire, detoxicate, and disperse congestion.

Indications: hot diseases, scabies, sore throat, pain in throat, scrofula, and carbuncles.

Notes: Experiments indicate that this herb can cool the blood and bring down blood pressure, bring down blood pressure by tonification, and reduce blood sugar.

CHINESE HERBS NAMED AFTER THEIR TASTES AND AROMAS

Herbs can be either sweet, sour, bitter, pungent, or salty—or a combination. Some are aromatic whereas others smell offensive.

Chinese: *Muxiang.* 木香

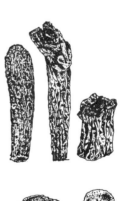

Re: 0703.

Common name: costusroot.

Family: Compositae.

Chinese name: wood aroma (so named because it is aromatic).

Scientific names: Aucklandia lappa Decne. and Saussurae lappa Clarke.

Pharmaceutical name: Radix Aucklandiae and Radix Saussureae.

Part used: dry root.

Dosage: 6 g.

Flavor: pungent.

Energy: warm.

Class: 11, herbs to regulate energy.

Meridians: lungs, liver, and spleen.

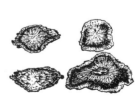

Actions: to promote energy circulation, relieve pain, and eliminate accumulations.

Indications: abdominal swelling and pain, diarrhea, and dysentery.

Notes: Experiments indicate that this herb can be effective in promoting

129

gastrointestinal peristalsis, can benefit the gallbladder and reduce jaundice, and can promote liver bile production and bile excretion.

Muxiang is a relatively strong herb for relieving energy stagnation in the stomach and intestine. It is often used to treat poor appetite, indigestion, and abdominal swelling and pain. It can be used with *huanglian* to treat diarrhea and tenesmus due to damp heat.

Chinese: *Xiaohuixiang.* 小茴香

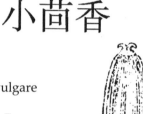

Re: 3306.
Common name: fennel.
Family: Umbelliferae.
Chinese name: fennel.
Scientific name: Foeniculum vulgare Mill.
Pharmaceutical name: Fructus Foeniculi.
Part used: ripe fruit.
Dosage: 2 to 5 g.
Flavor: pungent.
Energy: warm.
Class: 4, herbs to reduce cold sensations inside the body.
Meridians: liver, kidneys, spleen, and stomach.

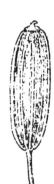

Actions: to promote energy flow, disperse congestion, warm up internal regions, and relieve pain.
Indications: hernia, pain in the lower abdomen, and intestinal rumbling.
Notes: This herb can warm the lower abdomen. It is most frequently used to treat only acute cases of cold abdominal pain in early stages.

Chinese: *Dingxiang.* 丁香
Re: 0026.
Common name: cloves.
Family: Myrtaceae.
Chinese name: T-shaped aroma (so named because its flowers are T-shaped and it's aromatic).
Scientific name: Eugenia caryophyllata Thunberg (Caryophyllus aromaticus L.).

130

Pharmaceutical name: Flos Caryophylli.
Part used: buds.
Dosage: 2 g.
Flavor: pungent.
Energy: warm.
Classes: herbs to regulate energy (class 11) and herbs to reduce cold sensations inside the body (class 4).
Meridians: lungs, spleen, stomach, and kidneys.

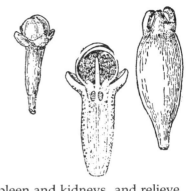

Actions: to bring down energy, warm up spleen and kidneys, and relieve pain.

Indications: hiccups, vomiting, spleen and kidney cold deficiency, and cold abdominal pain.

Notes: Experiments indicate that *dingxiang* is effective as a digestive and for promoting gastrointestinal peristalsis. It warms the spleen and stomach, and is good for cold stomach and hiccups due to cold.

Chinese: *Chouwutong.* 臭梧桐
Re: 3886.
Common name: forked clerodendron leaf.
Family: Verbenaceae.
Chinese name: stinky Chinese parasol tree (so named because of its offensive smell).
Scientific name: Clerodendron trichotomum Thunb.
Pharmaceutical name: Folium Clerodendri Trichotomi.
Parts used: young branches and leaves.
Dosage: 10 to 20 g.
Flavor: bitter and sweet.
Energy: cold.
Class: 3, herbs to counteract rheumatism.
Meridians: undetermined.

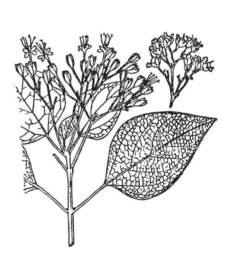

Actions: to clear heat, benefit water, expel wind and dampness, relieve pain, and reduce blood pressure.

131

Indications: blood in stools, suppression of urination, arthritis, lumbago and pain in legs, and hypertension.

Notes: Experiments indicate that *chouwutong* is an effective herb for relief of pain. It is an antirheumatic herb, and is also generally effective in reducing blood pressure.

Chinese: *Kushen.* 苦參

Re: 2624.

Common name: bitter sophora.

Family: Leguminosae.

Chinese name: bitter ginseng (so named due to its taste).

Scientific name: Sophora flavescens Ait.

Pharmaceutical name: Radix Sophorae Flavescentis.

Part used: root.

Dosage: 6 to 12 g.

Flavor: bitter.

Energy: cold.

Class: 2, herbs to reduce excessive heat inside the body.

Meridians: heart, spleen, and kidneys.

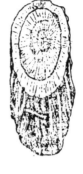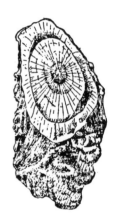

Actions: to clear up heat, dry up dampness, benefit water, destroy worms, and relieve itch.

Indications: diarrhea, dysentery, urination difficulty, scabies, and trichomonas vaginitis.

Notes: Experiments indicate that *kushen* can produce three effects: (1) It can promote urination, (2) it can be used for various types of cancer, and (3) it can be used as an antibacterial herb.

Although *kushen* is good for many symptoms, it is used mostly for external applications, because it is cold and bitter and can be harmful to weak patients. When *kushen* is used for internal consumption, it is usually combined with other herbs, such as *muxiang, gancao, danggui,* and *chishaoyao,* all of which are discussed in this book.

External applications of *kushen* are often used to treat eczema, furuncles, and carbuncles, as well as genital itch in women.

Chinese: *Kulianpi.* 苦楝皮

Re: 2658.

Common name: Chinaberry tree bark.

132

Family: Meliaceae.

Chinese name: bitter Chinaberry tree bark (so named due to its taste).

Scientific names: Melia toosendan Sieb. et Zucc. and Melia azedarach L.

Pharmaceutical name: Cortex Meliae.

Part used: white root bark.

Dosage: 10 to 15 g.

Flavor: bitter.

Energy: cold.

Class: 18, herbs to expel or destroy parasites.

Meridians: undetermined.

Actions: to destroy worms.

Indications: roundworms and hookworms.

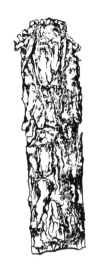

Chinese: *Suanzaoren.*

Re: 5292.

酸棗仁

Common name: jujube.

Family: Rhamnaceae.

Chinese name: sour date (so named because its fruits resemble dates and taste sour).

Scientific name: Ziziphus spinosa Hu.

Pharmaceutical name: Semen Ziziphi Spinosae.

Part used: kernel.

Dosage: 10 g.

Flavor: sweet.

Energy: neutral.

Class: 14, herbs to reduce anxiety.

Meridians: heart, liver, and gallbladder.

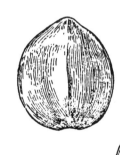
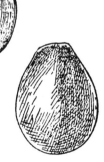

Actions: to secure the heart, calm down the spirits, check perspiration, and produce fluids.

Indications: insomnia, palpitations, forgetfulness, and deficiency perspiration.

Notes: Experiments indicate that *suanzaoren* can sedate and inhibit. *Suanzaoren* can be used to treat insomnia due to anxiety by nourishing the blood and the liver.

133

Chinese: *Xixin.* 細辛

Re: 3082.

Common name: Chinese wild ginger.

Family: Aristolochiaceae.

Chinese name: Fine and pungent (so named because its roots are very fine and taste pungent).

Scientific names: Asarum heterotropoides Fr. Schmidt var. mandshuricum (Maxim.) Kitag and Asarum sieboldii Miq.

Pharmaceutical name: Herba Asari.

Parts used: root and rhizoma.

Dosage: 5 g.

Flavor: pungent.

Energy: warm.

Class: 1, herbs to induce perspiration.

Meridians: heart, lungs, liver, and kidneys.

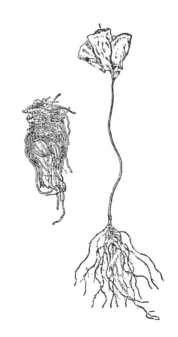

Actions: to expel cold, disperse wind, promote flow of water, and open up cavities.

Indications: headache due to wind dampness, asthma, cough, and rheumatism.

Notes: Experiments indicate that *xixin* is an effective herb for relief of pain, and it contains volatile oils. Since *xixin* is a relatively strong herb, it is particularly good at opening cavities to relieve pain. It disperses wind cold in the heart and the kidneys in particular. It is most often used to treat headache due to the common cold, body pain and nasal congestion due to external attack and yang deficiency, and fever with severe fear of cold.

CHINESE HERBS NAMED AFTER THEIR SHAPES

Many herbs are named after their shapes, such as cow's knee, dog's spine, and hundred parts.

Chinese: *Taizishen.* 太子参

Re: 0749.

Common name: root of heterophylly falsestarwort.

Family: Caryophyllaceae.

134

Chinese name: prince ginseng (so named because its roots resemble a fat prince).

Scientific name: Pseudostellaria heterophylla (Miq.) Pax ex Pax et Hoffm.

Pharmaceutical name: Radix Pseudostellariae.

Part used: tuberous root.

Dosage: 6 to 10 g.

Flavor: sweet and bitter.

Energy: slightly warm.

Class: 16, herbs to correct deficiencies.

Meridians: spleen and lungs.

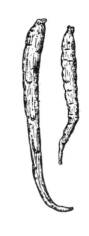

Actions: to tone up energy, benefit spleen, and produce fluids.

Indications: energy deficiency of spleen and stomach, lungs, energy deficiency, shortness of breath, asthma, cough, and thirst.

Notes: Experiments indicate that this herb is effective in treating various types of cancer.

Taizishen can tonify energy to treat fatigue and shortness of breath. It can also tonify yin, produce fluids, and quench thirst.

Chinese: *Niuxi*. 牛膝

Re: 0833.

Common names: two-toothed amaranthus and root of two-toothed achyranthes.

Family: Amaranthaceae.

Chinese name: cow's knee (so named because its stalks resemble the knees of a cow).

Scientific name: Achyranthes bidentata Bl.

Pharmaceutical name: Radix Achyranthis Bidentatae.

Part used: roots.

Dosage: 10 g.

Flavor: bitter and sour.

Energy: neutral.

Class: 12, herbs to regulate blood.

Meridians: liver and kidneys.

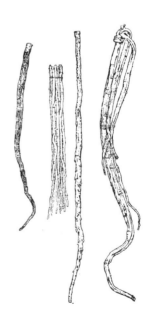

Actions: to activate blood and facilitate menstrual flow (raw), and to tone up liver and kidneys (processed).

Indications: suppression of menstruation, abdominal obstructions, headache due to liver fire, and pain in bones.

Notes: Experiments indicate that this herb can bring down blood pressure by tonification.

Chinese: *Gouji.* 狗脊
Re: 2949.

Common name: rhizome of East Asian tree fern.

Family: Dicksoniaceae.

Chinese name: dog's spine (so named because it looks like a dog's spine).

Scientific name: Cibotium barometz (L.) J. Sm.

Pharmaceutical name: Rhizoma Cibotii.

Part used: rhizome.

Dosage: 5 to 25 g.

Flavor: bitter and sweet.

Energy: warm.

Classes: herbs to counteract rheumatism (class 3) and herbs to correct deficiencies (class 16).

Meridians: liver and kidneys.

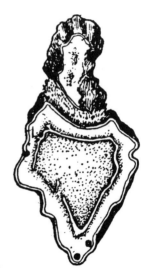

Actions: to tone up the liver and kidneys, strengthen the loins and legs, and remove wind and dampness.

Indications: lumbago, weak legs, enuresis, frequent urination, whitish vaginal discharge, and chronic ulcers.

Notes: This herb is effective for treating pain in the spine due to an accumulation of cold and dampness.

Chinese: *Gouteng.* 鈎藤
Re: 3436.

Common name: gambir.

Family: Rubiaceae.

Chinese name: hooky branches (so named because this herb has thorns like so many hooks).

Scientific names: Uncaria rhynchophylla (Miq.) Jacks, Uncaria macrophylla

136

Wall., Uncaria hirsuta Havil., Uncaria sinensis (Oliv.) Havil., and Uncaria sessilifructus Roxb.

Pharmaceutical names: Ramulus Uncariae Cum Uncis and Rhynchophylla.

Part used: branches.

Dosage: 10 g.

Flavor: sweet.

Energy: slightly cold.

Classes: herbs to reduce anxiety (class 14) and herbs to stop involuntary movements (class 15).

Meridians: liver and pericardium.

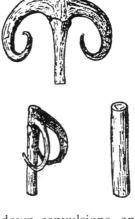

Actions: to stop wind, remove heat, calm down convulsions, and stop dizziness.

Indications: convulsions in children, dizziness, headache, fever, and twitching.

Notes: Experiments indicate that this herb can reduce anxiety and blood pressure, sedate and inhibit, and counteract epilepsy and convulsions. *Gouteng* is an ideal herb for light cases of convulsions at the beginning stage.

Chinese: *Zhuling.* 猪苓

Re: 4545.

Common name: umbellate pore fungus.

Family: Polyporaceae.

Chinese name: pig's fungus (so named because it is as black as pig dung, and it grows on trees like a fungus).

Scientific name: Polyporus umbellatus (Pers.) Fries.

Pharmaceutical name: Polyporus Umbellatus (Grifola).

Part used: fungus nucleus.

Dosage: 10 g.

Flavor: sweet.

Energy: neutral.

Class: 5, herbs to reduce dampness in the body.

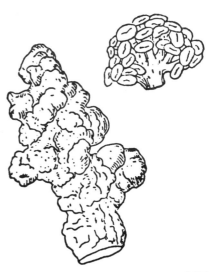

137

Meridians: kidneys and bladder.

Actions: to seep and benefit dampness.

Indications: diminished urination, edema, beriberi, urinary strains, and vaginal discharge.

Notes: Experiments indicate that this herb can promote urination.

Chinese: *Chuanwutou.* 川烏斗

Re: 0456.

Common name: monkshood.

Family: Ranunculaceae.

Chinese name: crow's head from Si Chuan (so named because it looks like the head of a crow, and the best quality of this herb is produced in Si Chuan).

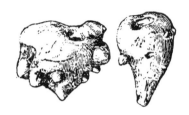

Scientific names: Aconitum chinense Paxton and Aconitum carmichaeli Debx.

Pharmaceutical name: Radix Aconiti.

Part used: tuberous root.

Dosage: 4 g.

Flavor: pungent.

Energy: hot.

Classes: herbs to counteract rheumatism (class 3) and herbs to reduce cold sensations inside the body (class 4).

Meridians: spleen, kidneys, and heart.

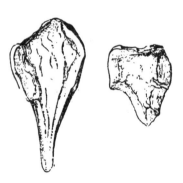

Actions: to remove wind and dampness, warm up meridians, disperse cold, and relieve pain.

Indications: acute rheumatic pain, spasms of arms and legs, paralysis of limbs, twitching and numbness, and cold headache.

Notes: Experiments indicate that this herb is effective for relief of pain. But it is extremely toxic when used in crude form, and needs to be processed in order to be safe for consumption.

Chinese: *Baibu.* 百部

Re: 1729.

Common name: wild asparagus.

Family: Stemonaceae.

Chinese name: hundred parts (so named because its roots are over one hundred in number).

138

Scientific names: Stemona sessilifolia (Miq.) Miq., Stemona japonica (Bl.) Miq., and Stemona tuberosa Lour.

Pharmaceutical name: Radix Stemonae.

Part used: tuberous root.

Dosage: 5 g.

Flavor: sweet and bitter.

Energy: slightly warm.

Class: 10, herbs to suppress cough and reduce sputum.

Meridians: lungs.

Actions: to lubricate lungs, suppress cough, bring down energy, and destroy worms.

Indications: cough due to deficiency fatigue, pulmonary tuberculosis, chronic bronchitis, and whooping cough.

Notes: Experiments indicate that *baibu* is effective for suppression of cough and it is also an antituberculotic herb.

CHINESE HERBS NAMED AFTER THEIR EFFECTS

Certain Chinese herbs are named for their particular effects. For instance, some are named after eye diseases, bone diseases, or wind diseases.

Chinese: *Gusuibu.*

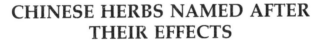

Re: 3421.

Common name: rhizome of fortune's drynaria.

Family: Polypodiaceae.

Chinese name: bone fracture remedy (so named due to its being effective for bone diseases).

Scientific names: Drynaria fortunei (Kunze) J. Sm. and Drynaria baronii (Christ) Diels.

Pharmaceutical name: Rhizoma Drynariae.

Part used: rhizome.

Dosage: 5 to 10 g.

Flavor: bitter.

Energy: warm.

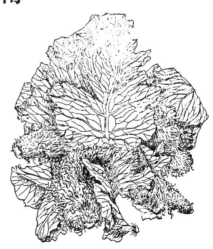

139

Classes: herbs to counteract rheumatism (class 3) and herbs to correct deficiencies (class 16).

Meridians: liver and kidneys.

Actions: to tone up the kidneys, connect tendons and bones, activate the blood, and relieve pain.

Indications: fracture, lumbago, and kidney deficiency with ringing in the ears.

Notes: This herb can tonify the kidneys to treat chronic diarrhea due to kidney deficiency. In addition, it can activate the blood and connect broken bones, which is why it can be used to treat fracture and pain in tendons and bones

Chinese: *Yuanzhi.* 遠志

Re: 2087.

Common name: slender-leaved milk-wort.

Family: Polygalaceae.

Chinese name: Long determination (so named because it is believed that by consuming this herb, one can develop the strong determination that goes a long way).

Scientific names: Polygala tenuifolia Willd. and Polygala sibirica L.

Pharmaceutical name: Radix Polyga-lae.

Part used: root.

Dosage: 5 g.

Flavor: bitter and pungent.

Energy: warm.

Class: 14, herbs to reduce anxiety.

Meridians: heart and kidneys.

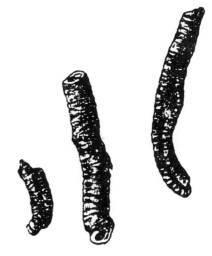

Actions: to calm down the spirits, benefit intelligence, transform sputum, open cavities, and disperse and eliminate.

Indications: insomnia, palpitations, forgetfulness, cough with copious sputum, carbuncles, and sore throat.

Notes: Experiments indicate that this herb is effective as an expectorant and it can sedate and inhibit. It contains saponin, which accounts for its being used as an expectorant.

140

Chinese: *Juemingzi, Caojueming.*

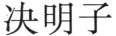

Re: 1906.

Common name: cassia seed.

Family: Leguminosae.

Chinese name: determining brightness seed (so named because it can sharpen vision).

Scientific names: Cassia obtusifolia L. and Cassia tora L.

Pharmaceutical name: Semen Cassiae.

Part used: ripe seeds.

Flavor: salty.

Energy: neutral.

Class: 2, herbs to reduce excessive heat inside the body.

Meridians: liver and kidneys.

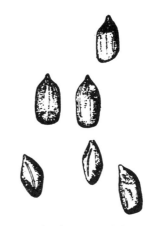

Actions: to clear up liver, benefit kidneys, expel wind, sharpen vision, and lubricate intestine for constipation.

Indications: headache due to hot liver, amaurosis, pinkeye with swelling, and discharge of dry stools with constipation.

Notes: Experiments indicate that this herb is generally effective in reducing blood pressure.

Chinese: *Fangfeng.* 防風

Re: 1985.

Common name: Chinese fangfeng.

Family: Umbelliferae.

Chinese name: wind-preventing herb (so named because this herb can counteract the attack of wind to prevent wind disease and stroke).

Scientific name: Ledebouriella divaricata (Turcz.).

Pharmaceutical name: Radix Ledebouriellae.

Part used: root.

Dosage: 5 g.

Flavor: pungent.

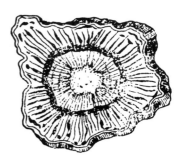

141

Energy: slightly warm.

Class: 1, herbs to induce perspiration.

Meridians: bladder, liver, lungs, spleen, and stomach.

Actions: to induce perspiration, disperse cold, relieve pain, and overcome dampness.

Indications: wind-dampness rheumatism.

Notes: Experiments indicate that *fangfeng* is effective for relief of pain and it is an antirheumatic herb. *Fangfeng* is good for excessive perspiration due to superficial deficiency and for prevention of the common cold.

Chinese: *Dafengzi.* 大楓子

Re: 0196.

Common name: chaulmoogra.

Family: Flacourtiaceae.

Chinese name: greater leprosy seed (so named because it can treat leprosy).

Scientific name: Hydnocarpus anthelmintica Pierre.

Pharmaceutical name: Semen Hydnocarpi.

Part used: ripe seeds.

Dosage: 2 to 4 g.

Flavor: pungent.

Energy: hot.

Class: 20, herbs for external applications.

Meridians: undetermined.

Actions: to expel wind, dry up dampness, attack poisons, and destroy worms.

Indications: scabies, boils, and leprosy.

Notes: *Dafengzi* is toxic.

CHINESE HERBS NAMED AFTER THEIR DISCOVERERS

Chinese: *Xuchangqing.* 徐長卿

Re: 3897.

Common name: root of paniculate swallowwort.

Family: Asclepiadaceae.

142

Chinese name: Mr. Xuchangqing (so named because it was discovered by him).

Scientific name: Cynanchum paniculatum (Bge.) Kitag.

Pharmaceutical name: Radix Cynanchi Paniculati.

Parts used: root and rhizome or whole plant with root.

Dosage: 3 to 10 g.

Flavor: pungent.

Energy: warm.

Class: 10, herbs to suppress cough and reduce sputum.

Meridians: undetermined.

Actions: to relieve pain, suppress cough, benefit water, reduce swelling, activate blood, and detoxicate.

Indications: stomachache, toothache, rheumatic pain, abdominal pain during menstruation, chronic tracheitis, and eczema.

Notes: Experiments indicate that *Xuchangqing* is effective for relief of pain and is also an antirheumatic herb. It is toxic and should be used cautiously by those with deficiency.

Chinese: *Luijinu.*
Re: 1897.

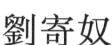

Common name: herb of diverse wormwood.

Family: Compositae.

Chinese name: Mr. Liujinu (so named because it was discovered by him).

Scientific names: Artemisia anomala S. Moore and Siphonostegia chinensis Benth.

Family: Scroplmlariaceae.

Pharmaceutical name: Herba Artemisiae Anomalae.

Part used: whole plant.

Dosage: 5 to 10 g.

Flavor: bitter.

Energy: warm.

Class: 12, herbs to regulate blood.

Meridians: heart and spleen.

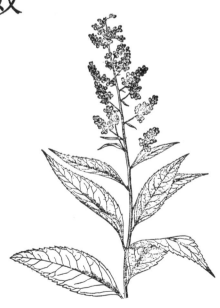

143

Actions: to activate the blood, relieve pain, and facilitate menstruation.

Indications: suppression of menstruation, pain due to blood coagulations, and injuries.

Chinese: *Duzhong.* 杜仲

Re: 2092.

Common name: eucommia bark.

Family: Eucommiaceae.

Chinese name: Du Zhong (so named because according to a Chinese legend, a person named Du Zhong made great intellectual achievements after taking this herb).

Scientific name: Eucommia ulmoides Oliv.

Pharmaceutical name: Cortex Eucommiae.

Part used: bark.

Dosage: 6 g.

Flavor: sweet and bitter.

Energy: warm.

Class: 16, herbs to correct deficiencies.

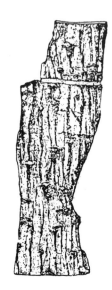

Meridians: liver and kidneys.

Actions: to tone up the liver and kidneys, strengthen tendons and bones, and secure fetus.

Indications: lumbago, fetus motion, kidney deficiency, headache and dizziness, and weak legs.

Notes: Experiments indicate that *duzhong* can bring down blood pressure by tonification, reduce blood fat, and be generally effective in reducing blood pressure.

CHINESE HERBS NAMED AFTER THEIR GROWING SEASONS

Some Chinese herbs are named after the season in which they are grown, including middle summer, winter-tolerating stem, and after-summer-see-me-not (which was discussed earlier).

Chinese: *Banxia.* 半夏

Re: 1550.

Common name: middle-summer pinellia.

144

Family: Araceae.

Chinese name: middle summer (so named because it grows in the middle of summer).

Scientific name: Pinellia ternata (Thunb.) Breit.

Pharmaceutical names: Rhizoma Pinelliae and Tuber Pinelliae.

Part used: rhizome.

Dosage: 8 g.

Flavor: pungent.

Energy: warm.

Classes: herbs to induce vomiting (class 7) and herbs to suppress cough and reduce sputum (class 10).

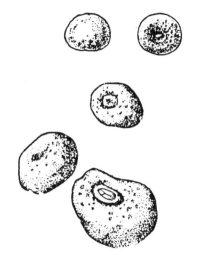

Meridians: spleen and stomach.

Actions: to dry up dampness, transform sputum, bring down upsurging energy, and relieve vomiting.

Indications: asthma, cough, vomiting, and external applications for carbuncles and swelling.

Notes: Experiments indicate that *banxia* is effective as an expectorant and can relieve vomiting.

Banxia in its raw form is toxic; it can cause sore throat, swollen tongue, and hoarseness, which is why it should be taken internally *only* after having been processed. According to a recent report, after it is decocted its toxic effects are substantially reduced. Nevertheless, pregnant women should use this herb with great care.

Chinese: *Rendongteng.* 忍冬藤

Re: 2417.

Common name: honeysuckle stem.

Family: Caprifoliaceae.

Chinese name: winter-tolerating stem (so named because this plant does not wither in the severe cold of winter).

Scientific name: Lonicera japonica Thunberg.

Pharmaceutical name: Caulis Lonicerae.

Part used: leafy stems.

Dosage: 11 to 33 g.

Flavor: sweet.

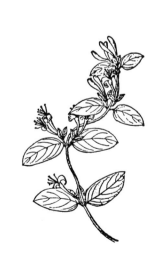

Energy: cold.

Class: 2, herbs to reduce excessive heat inside the body.

Meridians: heart and lungs.

Actions: to clear and detoxicate, and open passages of meridians.

Indications: fever in warm diseases, dysentery with blood in stools, contagious hepatitis, carbuncles, and pain in tendons and bones.

Notes: Experiments indicate that this herb is effective for various types of cancer.

Chinese: *Nuzhenzi.*
Re: 0467.

女貞子

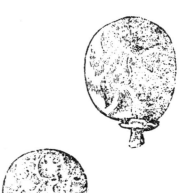

Common name: wax tree.

Family: Oleaceae.

Chinese name: winter green or chastity seed (so named because the leaves of this plant remain green in the severe cold of winter, which is comparable to a woman remaining faithful to her lover).

Scientific name: Ligustrum lucidum Ait.

Pharmaceutical name: Fructus Ligustri Lucidi.

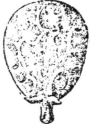

Part used: ripe fruit.

Dosage: 10 to 15 g.

Flavor: sweet and bitter.

Energy: neutral.

Class: 16, herbs to correct deficiencies.

Meridians: liver and kidneys.

Actions: to nourish yin, and tone up liver and kidneys.

Indications: liver-kidney yin deficiency, dizziness, seminal emission, and palpitations.

Notes: Experiments indicate that this herb is an effective heart tonic. In addition, *nuzhenzi* can tonify the kidneys and sharpen vision, and it is an effective herb for dizziness, ringing in the ears, and premature grey hair due to liver and kidney deficiency.

CHINESE FLOWERING HERBS

Flowers are a symbol of beauty; people appreciate their appealing colors and aromas. But many people do not realize that most flowers are also Chinese herbs.

*   *   *

146

Once upon a time, a goddess threw a party for her seven daughters. In the food she cooked, she used seven flowers, with one flower for each daughter. As a result, all her seven daughters grew up to be beautiful women, and remained beautiful and youthful forever. The seven daughters were so happy about the wonderful effects of the flowers that they begged their mother to do the same for women in the mundane world so that they too would remain beautiful forever. And so, the goddess ordered her seven daughters to plant flowers on earth for the women in the mundane world, which is why most flowers in Chinese medicine are good for women's disorders.

Chinese: *Hehuanhua.* 何歡花

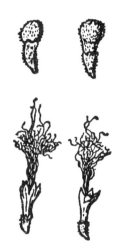

Re: 1880.
Common name: silk-tree flower.
Family: Leguminosae.
Chinese name: meeting-happiness flower.
Scientific name: Albizzia julibrissin Durazz.
Pharmaceutical name: flos Albiziae.
Part used: flower or bud.
Dosage: 3 to 10 g.
Flavor: sweet.
Energy: neutral.
Class: 14, herbs to reduce anxiety.
Meridians: heart and spleen.
Actions: to relax liver, regulate energy, and secure spirits.
Indications: congested chest, insomnia, forgetfulness, wind-fire eye diseases, blurred vision, sore throat, carbuncles, and injuries from falls.

Chinese: *Lianhua.* 蓮花

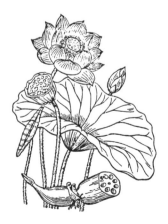

Re: 3693.
Common name: lotus flower.
Family: Nymphaceae.
Chinese name: lotus flower.
Scientific name: Nelumbo nucifera Gaertn.
Pharmaceutical name: Flos Nelumbinis.
Part used: flower.
Dosage: 5 to 10 g.
Flavor: bitter and sweet.
Energy: warm.
Class: 12, herbs to regulate blood.

Meridians: heart and liver.

Actions: to activate the blood, arrest bleeding, and remove dampness and wind.

Indications: vomiting of blood due to injuries from falls, eczema, and carbuncles.

Chinese: *Puhuang.* 蒲黄

Re: 5126.

Common name: cattail pollen.

Family: Typhaceae.

Chinese name: cattail pollen.

Scientific names: Typha angustifolia L. and Typha orientalis Presl.

Pharmaceutical name: Pollen Typhae.

Part used: pollen.

Dosage: 3 to 10 g.

Flavor: sweet.

Energy: neutral.

Class: 12, herbs to regulate blood.

Meridians: liver, spleen, and pericardium.

Actions: to disperse coagulation when used fresh, and arrest bleeding when fried.

Indications: menstrual pain due to blood coagulation, pain due to injuries causing blood coagulation, sore throat, and bleeding.

Notes: Experiments inducate that *puhuang* is an effective coagulant and can arrest bleeding (as a hemostatic). In addition, *puhuang* is good for irregular menstruation, acute pain in the lower abdomen, and dizziness.

Chinese: *Juhua.* 槐花

Re: 4127.

Common name: mulberry-leaved chrysanthemum.

Family: Compositae.

Chinese name: peak flower of September (so named because the flower of this plant reaches its peak in September and should be picked at that time).

Scientific name: Chrysanthemum morifolium Ramat.

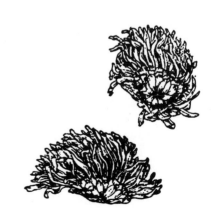

148

Pharmaceutical name: Flos Chyrsanthemi.
Part used: dry inflorescence.
Dosage: 8 g.
Flavor: sweet and bitter.
Energy: cool.
Class: 1, herbs to induce perspiration.
Meridians: lungs, liver, and kidneys.
Actions: to induce perspiration, clear heat, clear liver, and detoxicate.
Indications: eye diseases, pain in ears, dizziness, carbuncles, swelling, and headache due to wind heat.

Notes: *Juhua* is good for dispersing wind heat in the liver and gallbladder meridians, and also in the ears and eyes; it is often used to treat pinkeye, pain in the ears, and vertigo, due to wind heat.

It is estimated that in China, there are several hundred varieties of this herb. However, only the four that follow are commonly used. Sweet *juhua,* which is yellowish, and is used to disperse wind and reduce fever; white *juhua,* which is drunk as tea, and is used to clear the liver and sharpen vision; aromatic *juhua,* which is white and aromatic, and is used to treat dizziness and twitching in warm-hot diseases; and wild *juhua,* which is used to clear heat and to detoxicate.

Chinese: *Meiguihua.* 玫瑰花

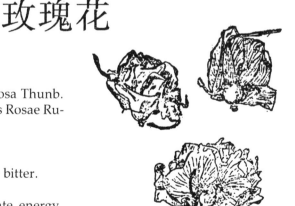

Re: 2483.
Common name: rose.
Family: Rosaceae.
Chinese name: rose.
Scientific name: Rosa rugosa Thunb.
Pharmaceutical name: Flos Rosae Rugosae.
Part used: flower.
Dosage: 3 to 6 g.
Flavor: sweet and slightly bitter.
Energy: warm.
Class: 11, herbs to regulate energy.
Meridians: liver and spleen.
Actions: to regulate energy, relieve energy congestion, harmonize the blood, and disperse blood coagulation.
Indications: energy pain in the liver and stomach, wind rheumatism, vomiting blood, discharge of blood from the mouth, irregular menstruation, vaginal discharge, dysentery, mastitis, and swelling.

Chinese: *Jiguanhua.* 鷄冠花
Re: 2451.
Common name: cockscomb.
Family: Amaranthaceae.
Chinese name: cockscomb.
Scientific name: Celosia cristata L.
Pharmaceutical name: Flos Celosiae Cristatae.
Part used: inflorescence.
Dosage: 5 to 10 g.
Flavor: sweet.
Energy: cool.
Classes: herbs to induce perspiration (class 1) and herbs to regulate blood (class 12).
Meridians: liver and kidneys.

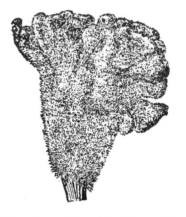

Actions: to cool blood and arrest bleeding.
Indications: hemorrhoids with discharge of blood, vomiting blood, coughing up blood, blood in urine, and vaginal bleeding and discharge.

Chinese: *Shegan.* 射干
Re: 3875.
Common name: blackberry lily.
Family: Iridaceae.
Chinese name: shooting dryness.
Scientific name: Belamcanda chinensis (L.) DC.
Pharmaceutical name: Rhizoma Belamcandae.
Part used: rhizome.
Dosage: 3 to 10 g.
Flavor: bitter.
Energy: cold.
Class: 2, herbs to reduce excessive heat inside the body.
Meridians: lungs and liver.

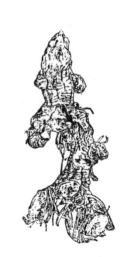

Actions: to clear up heat, counteract toxic effects, bring down energy, expel sputum, disperse blood, and heal swelling.
Indications: sore throat with swelling, cough, and carbuncles.
Notes: Experiments indicate that this herb is effective as an expectorant and can inhibit influenza. This herb is slightly toxic.

150

Chinese: *Danshen.* 丹參
Re: 0977.
Common name: purple sage.
Family: Labiatae.
Chinese name: red ginseng (so named because it is red and is shaped like ginseng).
Scientific name: Salvia miltiorrhiza Bge.
Pharmaceutical name: Radix Salviae Miltiorrhizae.
Part used: root.
Dosage: 10 g.
Flavor: bitter.
Energy: slightly cold.
Class: 12, herbs to regulate blood.
Meridians: heart and liver.

Actions: to activate the blood, regulate menstruation, clear up heat, and cool the blood.

Indications: irregular menstruation, suppression of menstruation, vaginal bleeding, abdominal obstructions, and insomnia.

Notes: Experiments indicate that this herb can produce seven effects. It can: (1) expand coronary arteries and prevent angina pectoris, (2) activate the blood and bring down blood pressure, (3) protect the liver, (4) soften and shrink the liver and the spleen, (5) increase red blood cells, (6) increase white blood cells, and (7) sedate and inhibit.

Chinese: *Chuipencao.* 垂盆草
Re: 1245.
Common name: weeping-plate plant.
Family: Crassulaceae.
Chinese name: stone nail (so named because it grows on cliffs with its leaves all over stones, and is shaped like a nail).
Scientific name: Sedum sarmento-sum Bge.
Pharmaceutical name: Herba Sedi Sarmentosi.
Part used: whole plant.
Dosage: 50 g.
Flavor: light, sweet, and slightly sour.

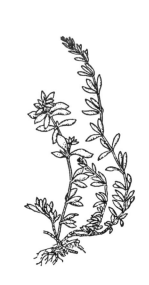

151

Energy: cool.
Class: 19, herbs for ulcers and tumors.
Meridians: undetermined.
Actions: to clear up heat, counteract toxic effects, heal swelling, and benefit water.
Indications: burns, carbuncles, snakebite, and cancerous swelling, particularly in liver cancer.

Chinese: *Huaihua.* 槐花
Re: 5078.
Common name: Japanese pagoda tree.
Family: Leguminosae.
Chinese name: Japanese pagoda flower.
Scientific name: Sophora japonica L.
Pharmaceutical name: Flos Sophorae.
Part used: buds.
Dosage: 6 to 15 g.
Flavor: bitter.
Energy: slightly cold.
Class: 12, herbs to regulate blood.
Meridians: liver and large intestine.
Actions: to sedate heat, cool the blood, and arrest bleeding.
Indications: hemorrhoids, discharge of blood from the anus, discharge of urine containing blood, nosebleeds, and dysentery.
Notes: Experiments indicate that this herb can produce four effects: (1) It can cool the blood and bring down blood pressure, (2) it can reinforce the resistance of capillary vessels, (3) it is an effective coagulant, and (4) it is generally effective in reducing blood pressure.

Chinese: *Mimenghua.* 密蒙花
Re: 4700.
Common name: butterfly bush.
Family: Loganiaceae.
Chinese name: dense-covered flower.

152

Scientific name: Buddleja officinalis Maxim.

Pharmaceutical name: Flos Buddlejae.

Part used: dried flowers or buds.

Dosage: 3 to 10 g.

Flavor: sweet.

Energy: cool.

Class: 2, herbs to reduce excessive heat inside the body.

Meridian: liver.

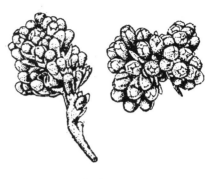

Actions: to expel wind, cool blood, lubricate liver, and sharpen vision.

Indications: pinkeye with swelling, watering of eyes, and amaurosis (optic atrophy).

Notes: *Mimenghua* is effective for nourishing the blood and sharpening the vision. It is good for those with liver-kidney yin deficiency and heat.

Chinese: *Jiegeng.* 桔梗

Re: 3642.

Common name: kikio root.

Family: Campanulaceae.

Chinese name: Solid and straight root (so named because the roots are straight and solid).

Scientific name: Platycodon grandiflorum (Jacq.) A.DC.

Pharmaceutical name: Radix Platycodi.

Part used: root.

Dosage: 6 g.

Flavor: pungent and bitter.

Energy: slightly warm.

Class: 10, herbs to suppress cough and reduce sputum.

Meridians: lungs.

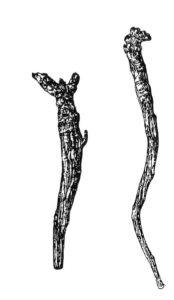

Actions: to expand lung energy, expel sputum, suppress cough, and drain off pus.

Indications: sore throat, hoarseness, cough and copious sputum, abscess of the lungs, suppurative pneumonia, and pulmonary gangrene.

Notes: Experiments indicate that this herb is effective as an expectorant, as it contains saponin.

153

Chinese: *Xuanfuhua.*
旋復花
Re: 4608.
Common name: innula flower.
Family: Compositae.
Chinese name: innula flower.
Scientific name: Inula japonica Thunb.
Pharmaceutical name: Flos Inulae.
Part used: flower head.
Dosage: 3 to 10 g.
Flavor: salty.
Energy: warm.
Class: 10, herbs to suppress cough and reduce sputum.
Meridians: lungs and large intestine.
Actions: to expel sputum, suppress cough, bring down energy, and calm down asthma.
Indications: cough, asthma, and hiccups.
Notes: *Xuanfuhua* is slightly toxic. It is good for internal obstruction of thick sputum with uprising energy.

Chinese: *Qianrihong.*
千日紅
Re: 0439.
Common name: flower of Globeamaranth.
Family: Amaranthaceae.
Chinese name: thousand-day red flower.
Scientific name: Gomphrena globosa L.
Pharmaceutical name: Flos Gomphrenae.
Part used: inflorescence or whole plant.
Dosage: 3 to 10 g (flower), 15 to 30 g (whole plant).
Flavor: sweet.
Energy: neutral.
Class: 12, herbs to regulate blood.
Meridians: undetermined.

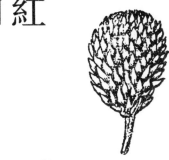

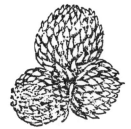

154

Actions: to clear liver, disperse congestion, relieve cough, treat asthma, and cool blood.

Indications: headache, cough, dysentery, whooping cough, scrofula, boils, eye pain due to hot liver, headache from hypertension, and chronic tracheitis.

Chinese: *Ziwan.* 紫菀

Re: 4866.

Common name: purple aster.

Family: Compositae.

Chinese name: purple-soft roots (so named because the roots are purple and soft).

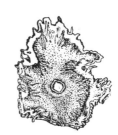

Scientific name: Aster tataricus L.f.

Pharmaceutical name: Radix Asteris.

Part used: root.

Dosage: 8 g.

Flavor: bitter.

Energy: warm.

Class: 10, herbs to suppress cough and reduce sputum.

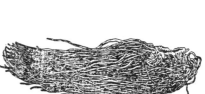

Meridians: lungs.

Actions: to warm up the lungs, expel sputum, suppress cough, and relieve asthma.

Indications: cough due to wind cold, asthma, and vomiting of blood in cough due to deficiency fatigue.

Notes: Experiments indicate that this herb is effective as an expectorant. It contains flavonone, which can act on the cardiovascular system, on the one hand, and arrest bleeding, suppress cough, and expel sputum, on the other.

GUIDE TO APPROXIMATE EQUIVALENTS

CUSTOMARY				METRIC
Ounces Pounds	Cups	Tablespoons	Teaspoons	Grams Kilograms
			¼ t.	1.25 g
			½ t.	2.5 g
			1 t.	5 g
			2 t.	10 g
½ oz.		1 T.	3 t.	15 g
1 oz.		2 T.	6 t.	30 g
2 oz.	¼ c.	4 T.	12 t.	60 g
4 oz.	½ c.	8 T.	24 t.	120 g
8 oz.	1 c.	16 T.	48 t.	240 g
1 lb.	2 c.			480 g
2 lb.	4 c.			
2.2 lb.				1 kg

Keep in mind that this is not an exact conversion, but generally may be used in measuring herbs.

156

INDEX

157

About the Author

Dr. Henry C. Lu received his Ph.D. from the University of Alberta, Edmonton, Canada. He taught at the University of Alberta and the University of Calgary between 1968 and 1971, and has practised Chinese medicine since 1972. Dr. Lu now teaches Chinese medicine by correspondence. His students live in many countries, including the United States, Canada, England, Australia, Sweden, Italy, Germany, France, New Zealand, Switzerland, Mexico, and Japan.

The author is best known for his translation of *Yellow Emperor's Classics of Internal Medicine* from Chinese into English, and for the Chinese College of Acupuncture and Herbology he established in Vancouver and Victoria, British Columbia, Canada, for the instruction of traditional Chinese medicine. Other Sterling books by the author are *Chinese System of Food Cures* and *Chinese Foods for Longevity*.

Dr. Lu has practised Chinese herbal medicine for over twenty years. He invented herbal formulas in powdered form for his patients at his Vancouver clinic, and teaches his students how to make these powdered formulas.

Dr. Lu lives in Surrey, British Columbia, with his wife, Janet, their son, Albert, and daughter, Magnus. Correspondence to Dr. Lu should be addressed to the Academy of Oriental Heritage, P.O. Box 8066, Blaine, WA U.S.A. 98230, or P.O. Box 35057, Station E, Vancouver, B.C., Canada V6M 4G1.